Praise for *Buddha and Einstein* ~~Walk Into a Bar~~

"I've known Guy as a dynamic, charismatic, and savvy presenter; now I know him as a clear and persuasive writer. His style is fresh, light, and bright. This book's positive outlook, clarity, and attention to detail will undoubtedly place it at the top of many a reading list."
– Prof. Erantha de Mel, PhD; author of *Optimizing the Infinite Mind*

"Guy's book is so unique, that after 40 years of practice as a psychotherapist I have put his ideas into practice, which have brought amazing results. This book will bring great insight to all who will read it and put these words and actions of wisdom into practice."
—Dr. Hans Vischjager, director of BEHA Institute
for Psychological Studies

"This book immediately captured my interest and enlightened me to the many possibilities of mankind, the impossible is possible! It is very refreshing and unique in its approach. I am sure the ICPT (International Council of Professional Therapists) would find it as interesting and as educational as I have."
—Helen Pourouna, ICPT director of operations;
editor of ICPT Magazine

"*Buddha and Einstein Walk Into a Bar* sounds like the start of a joke and Guy admits this right up front. But this is a serious book that ties modern science with deep philosophy. It talks about dark matter and string theory and quantum mechanics and also about how neuroplasticity makes it possible for our brains to be constantly evolving and adapting. Even better, Guy shows you how to consciously channel that adapting so that each day you are more able to achieve what you would like to while also ridding yourself of the tension that is so much a part of our lives."
—Srikumar Rao, PhD, Columbia Business School professor (ret.);
author of *Happiness at Work*

BUDDHA AND EINSTEIN WALK INTO A BAR

HOW NEW DISCOVERIES ABOUT MIND, BODY, AND ENERGY CAN HELP INCREASE YOUR LONGEVITY

GUY JOSEPH ALE

President, Lifespan Seminar®
Vice President, Asia Pacific Association of Psychology

This edition first published in 2018 by New Page Books,
an imprint of Red Wheel/Weiser, LLC

With offices at:
65 Parker Street, Suite 7
Newburyport, MA 01950
www.redwheelweiser.com
www.newpagebooks.com

ISBN: 978-1-63265-140-2

Library of Congress Cataloging-in-Publication
Data available upon request.

Cover design by *the*bookdesigners
Main cover image by intueri/shutterstock
Silhouette figures by bluedog studio/shutterstock and grynold/
shutterstock
Interior by PerfecType, Nashville, Tennessee
Typeset in Adobe Garamond Pro and DIN OT

Printed in Canada
MAR
10 9 8 7 6 5 4 3 2 1

To Teresa, for your heart and mind.

CONTENTS

Part I: Personal Background

Part II: Scientific and Spiritual Foundations

Part III: Mastering the Mind and Body

Part IV: Everyday Applications

PART ONE

Personal Background

CHAPTER ONE

BADLEM

Buddha and Einstein walk into a bar. They meet inside with Alexander the Great, Darwin, Lincoln, and Nelson Mandela. It's their monthly meeting. In each of these meetings one person suggests a topic of discussion. Everyone orders drinks, and because it's Einstein's turn to introduce a topic, he says, "There's this gentleman in Los Angeles, California, named Guy Joseph Ale, who has been researching since 1992 the proposition that we humans have a latent capacity to sense how long we can live. I would like him today to explain his findings." The others nod in agreement and Einstein says, "Guy, the floor is yours."

Thank you, Albert. Gentlemen. This book would not exist if I hadn't almost died from a lower back emergency in 2007. I explain this in detail later in the book, but for now I'll just say that being that close to death prompted me to ask myself: What is the biggest understanding I have at this point about myself and life? The clear answer that came back was that I'd known since 1992 how long I could live. I've devoted my life since then to researching the scientific, spiritual, behavioral, and evolutionary aspects of this awareness and its myriad implications in everyday life.

The simplest analogy of knowing how long you can live is having a fuel gauge in your vehicle of flesh, blood, and bones. You can go through life without knowing how much energy is in your tank, just like early vehicles could drive without fuel gauges. However, developing fuel gauges in later models clearly gave drivers better control of their cars.

I realize, gentlemen, that you all represent different parts of my own psyche, the dominant instincts driving me through life. Each one of you gave me guidance along the way. The phrases you communicated would vary slightly at different times, but each of you transmitted a clear message according to what your characters and work exemplify.

Buddha spoke of self-knowledge: Understand yourself and trust yourself.

Alexander communicated: You live only this once; you can.

Darwin stressed an intellectual grasp of this awareness, first to understand it on my own, and then to explain it to others.

Lincoln had a singular repeating instruction: How does it benefit others?

Einstein focused on imagination: Anything that is based in reason and facts is possible.

Mandela stressed pragmatism and responsibility, for what this awareness means in my own life, and for seeing it through to a broader communication.

How does this guidance happen? In several ways. For example, I would go to bed, even last night, a fifty-eight-year-old boy dreaming, and would ask for support. The nickname acronym for all your names is **BADLEM.** Sometimes one of you would speak up, and sometimes I'd hear a group voice.

I would say, "Please help me." And BADLEM would respond: "We are helping you. Breathe. Don't rush. We are guiding you."

Or, BADLEM would ask, "Will you accept this job?"

I have no choice. I can't not do it.

Or, during my twice-weekly swims, which are great meditation sessions, we would have a conversation. Here are a few versions of these talks:

Mandela: "It always seems impossible until it's done. If you can maintain your faith in the soundness and viability of this vision, your anxieties and impatience melt away. You gain a larger perspective on your life, and a deeper authority and responsibility to realize this promise of 102 years (the duration that I sense I can live). There is no passion to be found playing small—in settling for a life that is less than the one you are capable of living."

Alexander: "Think outside of the box. Don't follow others' examples but find your own path. Find a way to accomplish what you see fit. You have the license."

BADLEM as a group voice: "Use our wisdom, imagination, and strength. It is possible. Trust yourself."

And Alexander again: "Do what others are unable or unwilling to do. That's what leaders do. This is how you inspire others."

Or: "Dear Albert, I heard that one of your students at Princeton once saw the little pocket notebook you carried around and asked, 'Professor Einstein, is that where you keep all your great ideas?' To which you replied, 'Great ideas? I've only ever had one.'" That is how I feel about sensing how long I can live. It is the deepest insight I've had about myself and life. Everything else is an interpretation of this awareness, and the framework that this perception puts on my life.

With all the intellectual and practical challenges of being alive, I know in my bones that I'm on the right track, living the life that I was meant to live. How do I know this? Because this is the best version of me at the present age of fifty-eight. This is where I'm aligned with health and longevity. If I had done anything differently last year, five years ago, or twenty-five years ago, I would not be at this precise point on my path through life, and would not be as healthy as I am. I'm operating from the premise that I can live another forty-five years, and everything I do fits into this vision. This keeps my anxieties at bay, fills me with hope and purpose, and enables me to find the balance between fun and work.

Darwin: "So you are proposing that once we develop deeper awareness of our mind and body, we can understand the amount of energy in our body?"

Yes. Naturally, this theory will be proven valid or false only when I reach the end of my life and see how long I'd lived. To state the obvious, there's no precedent when we do something completely new. I derived my strength and conviction in this belief by talking with each one of you along the road. Each of you replied to my inquiries: Is it possible? Am I on solid ground? Am I not a fool? But when all is said and done, it boils down to a humble, strong, slap-in-the-butt simple reality; it comes down to the basic formula of life: eat well, sleep well, treat yourself and others well. If you do this, and continue breathing freely at every moment, you are exactly where you need to be, headed precisely where you need to go.

Einstein speaks: "Trust your intuition. The only source of knowledge is experience. I never made one of my discoveries through the process of rational thinking."

Buddha, the elder statesman of the group, looks at the others and says, "We want this awareness brought forward. We have given you this job because we know that you can do it. The path exists, and you are on it. Trust yourself and trust your mind and body, so you can benefit from this awareness and explain it to others." He brings the meeting to an end: "This is your journey through life. This is your path through existence. You will live 102 years, balancing the world inside you with the world outside. You will enjoy life as much as possible, making the biggest contribution in the world through what you think and how you act. You'll arrive at your deathbed a wise old man, and then the door will open and you will pass through."

Dear reader, the purpose of this book is to present the clearest, most comprehensive current record of the spiritual and scientific discoveries that enable us to sense how long we can live, and to give you practical tools to live your longest and healthiest life.

To help you achieve this higher mastery of your mind, body, and energy, we will go on a grand spiritual and mental adventure of cosmic dimensions while keeping your feet firmly on the ground. We will first go out into the universe at large and then bring that large universe back into your body.

We will describe the latest discoveries in new cosmology, neuroplasticity, superstring theory, and epigenetics to show that the consciousness animating the cosmos informs every cell in the human body. Simply put, when we access our innate intuition, we access universal intelligence.

Once the theory has been clearly explained we will move into practice, because understanding how long we can live is only the first part of the equation. The other crucial part is acquiring the self-management skills that enable us to realize that potential. I will provide step-by-step descriptions of my organization's (Lifespan Seminar) multiple-award-winning techniques, including stress management, good nutrition, sufficient rest, and active lifestyle that will help you to live your best life.

CHAPTER TWO

Formative Years

I am now a proud American citizen, but I was born in Georgia, which at the time was part of the Soviet Union, and although I spent only eight of my fifty-eight years in that country, I still carry a clear Georgian identity inside. Georgians are reputed to be fiercely independent, and that trait appeals to my own sense of individuality and freedom. The folk tales tell of people in the Caucasus Mountains living well past one hundred years. But current studies do not support those legends. There are in the world Blue Zones, areas where there is documented evidence of high percentages of living centenarians (persons one hundred years and older), and super-centenarians (persons 110 and over), and Georgia is not one of them. These Blue Zones are Icaria, Greece; Loma Linda, California; Nicoya Peninsula, Costa Rica; Okinawa, Japan; and Sardinia, Italy.

Nonetheless, because of Georgia's pleasant climate and history, being at the crossroads of religions and civilizations that have passed through and influenced its ways of life, it was regarded as the bread-basket of the entire region, and its bountiful cuisine and joyous food culture are well-known and widely appreciated. I gained from this healthy eating habits for a lifetime: a love of fruits and vegetables, and an instinctive understanding of what makes for good nutrition—to begin with, the opposite of fast food.

When I was four, our family moved to Uzbekistan, in Central Asia, and I lived there until the age of eight. Uzbekistan has a desert climate, and temperatures can reach triple digits in the summer. When I was eight we went back to Georgia for another four years. My parents divorced, and when I was twelve years old, our family, which consisted of my mother, sister, grandmother, and me, moved to Israel. Looking back, it is clear that my parents' divorce was a big factor in my rebelliousness and experimentation in the years following. I didn't have a father figure in my life, someone to set clear boundaries, and there were basic things I had to figure out on my own, which on the one hand creates a sense of uncertainty, but on the other a sense of liberation.

These early experiences in diverse countries and cultures ingrained in me the awareness that there is no one "correct" way of doing things. People in Georgia, Uzbekistan, Israel, and other places I've lived and visited go about their lives in different ways—and all of these ways work. This realization gives our psyche a sense of flexibility and of limitless possibilities, and the license to think outside of boundaries. We humans set designations on ourselves, define ourselves as an American, an executive, a blonde, a poor athlete, not good at math, and so forth—and through these descriptions we put borders on our minds and lives.

Question everything, even the need for questioning.

Nothing is right for you but what your own heart says.

I was born into a Jewish family, lived in a Muslim country as a child, and have lived in predominantly Christian societies as an adult. I have never felt a part of any one religion, and have always felt at one with God.

I have only two recollections of my father from my entire life before he left our family for good.

Mental snapshot: I'm about six years old. We are living in Samarkand, Uzbekistan. I am awoken in the middle of the night. There are strangers in our house (KGB men, I later found out) searching our home—for what? They're silent and efficient, routinely going from room to room, flinging open cupboards, drawers, closets. They turn our home upside down, take Father with them, and leave. What were they looking for? I've never found out.

Mental snapshot: I'm eight years old at my grandma's home in Kutaisi, Georgia. Father is being abusive toward my mom, not physically but mentally, berating her at length, and Mom is crying. I feel helpless. I go over and put my arms around Mom. We are family: mom, grandma, sister, and me; and he, Father, is a harmful presence who doesn't fit in this unit.

These are the two memories that Father left behind. But we never talked about him much. The unspoken sense was "good riddance."

Grandma's house is worth mentioning for several reasons. This was our extended family's headquarters, where all my cousins, our own little family, and everyone else who was drawn into Grandma's generous orbit willingly gravitated. We kids considered this home the most wonderful place in the world, filled with comfort, safety, treats, and warmth, all of which left us with a sense of belonging and unconditional love for our entire life.

Our stay in this home is notable for one other unforgettable occurrence: The house stood on a hill overlooking a river named Rioni, which literally translates to "river." When the river was at an ebb, which was most of the time, you could cross to the other bank with water reaching only up to your knees. Then, with what seemed to my young mind as no prior notice, the water would surge. A dam upriver would open, the river would swell, and you'd see a drowning person carried downstream. Imagine witnessing on a regular basis the horrifying sight of a person's head bobbing in and out of the water as they're being washed in the current. Grandma's living room windows overlooked the river, and once every few months we would hear loud shrieks, rush to the window, and watch another man (these were all men's voices) drowning. We would see a head dipping in the water, rise out with choking cries, and disappear back in. This spectacle lasted approximately thirty seconds to a minute at a time before the victim was overpowered by the current. And then silence. The river kept flowing. Life went on.

Near-Death Experiences

I was nearly killed riding a motorcycle when I was seventeen. I was knocked off my bike from behind by a speeding car on a highway. Commonly in situations like this, certain images crystallize in our minds and stay there forever. I have a clear recollection of lying on my back in the middle of the four-lane highway, my helmeted head facing the oncoming traffic. Instinctively, I rolled to the left and off the road and was saved. When an incident like this happens, there naturally is a humble recognition of the precarious nature of existence. In a very real sense, you've gained a whole new appreciation for life, because you have seen what it would be like to almost lose it.

My second brush with physical death happened in 2007 when I underwent back surgery. As the surgeon explained, a disk fragment in my lower back broke off the edge of a vertebra and lodged itself in the nerve canal. As I attempted to move my limbs, this bone chip in the spinal canal touched on the nerve endings and sent piercing signals to the brain. I could not walk, stand, sit, or move my body while lying without debilitating pain. I understood at this time what it meant to be totally incapacitated.

Following an ordeal that lasted several weeks, while the true nature of my situation was being diagnosed and the appropriate treatment determined, I went into surgery and then physical rehabilitation, and came out whole as ever, now with an exceptional perspective on the tenuous character of the human body.

If health is not there, nothing is there.

Your life can be at the best circumstances imaginable: You can have someone you love who loves you back; you can have a happy family; you can have wealth and success at work and in society. All this abundance notwithstanding, an incident like this strips your existence down to its essence. *Can I move my left leg, can I lift the comforter off my body, can I get off the bed, will I be able to stand?* The simple act of relieving yourself, which your mind remembers having done many times effortlessly and routinely, becomes a series of small but enormous challenges, each suffused with excruciating pain.

Will I be able to take care of myself? Will I be able to maintain my dignity, to not be a burden to others? When the entire experience was over, it seemed that I'd lost my life and gained it back.

To revisit my teenage years, the first place we lived upon arrival in Israel was Nazareth, and then I lived three years on a kibbutz (communal farm) near the Jordanian border. Later I joined my mother when she moved to Tel Aviv, and at eighteen I enlisted into military service alongside all my peers. Things came to a head when I inadvertently nearly killed three people in two separate traffic incidents.

Hell came calling on me at age twenty-five. It first knocked on my door four years earlier, knocked me off my feet for several months, but I regained balance and kept walking, oblivious to the full severity of the blow. From that close distance, how could I have known otherwise? But first things first.

I was twenty-one, serving in the Israeli Defense Force (IDF), mandatory for all men and women. My paratroop unit was stationed in the field for live-fire exercises, and on that glorious afternoon I was driving a large open vehicle (a "command car," in army-speak) to a nearby base to get supplies. In the passenger seat was my friend and fellow soldier Batya (not a girlfriend, but a good friend). We had cleared the dirt path and were driving on a paved road still in the woods, gorgeous scenery, not a soul or even another car around. We were joking and laughing, with the warm wind whipping through our hair.

The road curved to the left at a mild angle before coming to a stop sign. I brought the vehicle to a full stop and turned my head toward Batya, and she wasn't there. I pulled the handbrake, jumped out, and went around to her side of the vehicle. She was on the asphalt unconscious, shaking uncontrollably, her head in a widening pool of blood. She'd fallen out of the vehicle as we took the curve in the road. At this time helmets and seatbelts were not required in command cars. In fact, using seatbelts was discouraged in occupied territories, because they would hinder your response if you came under sudden assault. Both seatbelts and helmets in open vehicles would be obligatory in IDF after this incident.

I radioed for an ambulance. Batya, still unconscious, was taken to a hospital, and I was put in standard detention for two weeks, as per army regulations for this type of accident, so MP investigators can have unrestricted access to the parties involved. Needless to say, I was very upset, walking in the brig as if in a haze. No one was blaming me; the commander of the unit visited me and brought regards from others, but the fact remained: I drove the vehicle, and Batya was fighting for her life. She recovered consciousness after a week but remained in critical condition, requiring several brain surgeries.

The investigation completed early, and I was released after ten days, cleared of any wrongdoing. I returned to the unit uncertain of the reception, but everyone was gracious toward me, the underlying sense being that bad things happen in life and this was one of them.

Batya recovered fully. She was granted an early discharge from the army on medical grounds, and was back to her bubbly, cheerful self, though a large scar on her skull indicated what she'd gone through. Her parents threw a big poolside party at a fancy hotel, and the entire unit was invited. I was well aware of my good fortune that Batya had survived. I mean, who wants to go through life with that kind of stain on their psyche?

Fast-forward to age twenty-five. I had just graduated from an acting academy, and had my first professional role in the musical *Odysinbad,* an adaptation of the stories of Odysseus and Sinbad the sailor, as part of the Youth and Children Theater. That night, at 6 p.m., was the gala performance.

I was in a relationship with lovely Leila, the most desirable woman I've ever met. Leila seemed a direct descendant of Sofia Loren and Ingrid Bergman, with their lush sensuality, and of Marlene Dietrich and Greta Garbo, with their ethereal mystique. She was alluring doing the most commonplace things. No one could avert their eyes when she entered a room. As she herself once aptly observed, I carried myself as a peacock when we walked hand in hand on the street.

When we first met, Leila was coming off a ten-year relationship with her high-school sweetheart. They still lived together, but she was looking for a new apartment while gently navigating the separation. They appeared to be on good terms, but Leila was obviously distressed, and because I was so smitten with her I resolved to be always available when she needed. It was revealed later (and I'm only sharing this because Leila is a fictitious name) that her boyfriend had slept with her sister, and this fact was present like an elephant in the room each time the entire family gathered at her parents' house. Leila and her sister weren't speaking. The atmosphere was depressing, with awkward attempts at lightness.

For this or other reasons Leila, the wild flower, had a thorny and venomous side. When she felt threatened, this beautiful creature would turn into a monster, slashing and thrashing at whatever came near her, angry at everything and everyone.

On the opening day of *Odysinbad,* at about 4 p.m. on a gorgeous Tel Aviv afternoon, Leila and I were driving to the theater. It was rush hour, with cars bunched up together and moving very slowly. We were at a red light and when it turned to green, I made a right turn going approximately 5 mph. Suddenly there was a thud on the windshield, the engine of my little Autobianchi cut, and the car stalled. I got out and went around to the passenger side, from where the impact came. Two old ladies were lying on the asphalt, unconscious in a widening pool of blood. Hell.

They were crossing the street and had come between cars. I didn't see them. They hit their heads on the windshield and then the asphalt. A big commotion ensued. We were in the shopping center of Tel Aviv and, Israelis being a garrulous kind, we were quickly surrounded by a crowd.

In severe crises like this, this my system kicks into autopilot: calm, pragmatic, analytic. The deed had been done, getting emotional was counterproductive; the focus shifted onto specific actions. Call an ambulance: Someone already had. Notify the theater: Tell them I'd be delayed. Stay and wait for ambulances and police. The ambulances arrived and took the still-unconscious ladies (one was seventy-two and the other seventy-four) to an emergency room. The police arrived and started collecting evidence.

The long and the short of it was that the opening show had to be cancelled. The lead actor couldn't make it, so 700 children, their parents, and their teachers had to be sent home.

I, my mother, and my sister took turns at the ladies' bedsides at the hospital while they were in comas. They teetered on the verge of death for ten long days before finally they both revived, but the earth under my feet shook for a lot longer. By the grace of God I wouldn't have to carry the burden of their deaths on my psyche forever, but I retreated into my "mental cave" and stayed there for a good six months. It was hell. What? Being out of control. Being not in charge of my life. When things—and by implication, bad things—keep happening to you and you are unable to stop them. You feel hopeless, helpless, puny, overwhelmed by forces larger than yourself; you are at their complete mercy.

I still attended to my obligations. There was the show to perform, rehearsals for a new show to begin, the relationship with Leila. But I drew inside myself, like an injured animal crawling into its lair licking its wounds. I looked at the ruins that were my present life: the unhealthy dynamics with Leila, my being completely subsumed in her needs and neglecting my own well-being; this last accident; feeling generally frustrated, adrift. The outcome of this lengthy wrenching process was that the tiger in me awoke. Raised its head from the slumber in which it had been, stretched lazily pawing the ground with its feet, let out a soft purr, which gradually grew into a deep roar, and said, "No, I don't like this one bit. I am made for much better things than this. This is not good enough for me."

I came to see this entire incident as a gift. I'd been taken to the abyss and made to look into it, and God said, "Is this what you want, my son?" I could see where I was headed if I kept on the path I was walking: impulsive, accident prone, and in unforgivable consequence of my recklessness, endangering other people's lives—a wretched, sleep-walking fool.

Profound grief and sublime joy are closely located feelings. Both strike at the center of your heart.

These two episodes crystallized into a single vision of the pair of warnings I'd received: You don't get another chance to be stupid. Two is enough. Three strikes and you're out. What do you do with this invaluable gift of having your eyes opened? You are deeply grateful. Now you know that one alternative to a good life is chaos.

I had gone to an acting academy in Tel Aviv, following which I had a professional contract with a theater company. But after visiting the afore-mentioned abyss I had a visceral realization—an epiphany, really—that the only way to be able to harness my energies and take control of my life was by pursuing my highest ambition and most sacred dream. Only then would I be able to sublimate the feelings of frustration at daily banalities into something beautiful and worthwhile. I decided to move to New York and pursue movie acting.

Some guys go to the Amazon jungle to test their mettle; I went to the jungle of New York—glorious, exciting, rough-and-tumble New York, where in the midst of one of the most crowded cities on the planet you can feel like the loneliest person in the world.

Live fearlessly, as if the whole world belongs to you, because it does.

Trials and Lessons

I lived as an illegal alien in New York for almost seven years. I knew from the start that the first order of business was to learn English. (I had been a very bad student, coming to the States with about fifty words in English.) We don't think about such a basic necessity when we go about our normal daily lives, but if you were dropped in a foreign city, such as Beijing, China, without the ability to communicate with other people to express your feelings, needs, knowledge, and identity, you would feel like something less than human. You might sometimes feel like a deaf-mute animal caged in its silence. Some foreigners upon arrival would gravitate toward their native enclaves—a French enclave, a Turkish enclave, or a Chinese enclave—and speak mainly in their native tongue, but that was never my intention. I wanted to become a part of this country and master English quickly. I read as much as I could, in a process I jokingly referred to as "carpet bombing." I would look up in dictionary every word I didn't know. After a few years it became apparent that I had acquired a much richer vocabulary than an average native speaker. I had looked up words such as *penultimate* and *misogynist* as often as I had looked up *desk* and *hose*. I didn't know how rare or common those words were; to me they were all unfamiliar. So once again, from a problem a benefit emerges: I am now a great lover and master of English, this flood of a language—the language of the rest of my life.

The trials of living as an illegal alien for almost seven years made me reach inside and discover resources I didn't know existed. The image is of a subterranean elevator going down. A crisis causes you to submerge to the bottom of your psyche in order to locate strength within yourself, and you feel you've reached the center of your being, where you are standing on solid ground and you can handle this situation. However, several months or years later, a new incident occurs that requires deeper resources from you, and, lo and behold, you discover you can go deeper than where you felt was your previous bottom, what you thought was your limit.

Here's a little ditty that appeared during those years: faith, focus, fun.
Faith in myself.
Focus on my goal.
Fun while I'm traveling this path.

Reflecting on the path I've traveled, and without diminishing the significance of the achievement, will I ever forget:

- Clawing and crawling my way into low-paying jobs only to be let go when my illegal status was discovered?
- Being unable to afford the littlest brush with the law for fear of being deported from the United States for good?
- Struggling with loneliness, alienation, and sense of belonging?

The most important lesson that remains from this experience is correct self-perception: Do I see myself as the ostensible facts of a particular situation might show me, and how the outside world might see me, or can I maintain a vision of myself that is not yet apparent to the outside world?

Gifts I give to myself are proud humility and humble pride: humility to do my job, and pride in knowing that I am second to none. Just as no one can give me a sense of honor if I don't first locate it in myself, so the greatest "achievements" in the world can't save me from despair if I don't know who I am. When the world saw me as a pauper, I saw myself as a prince.

Dear reader, the purpose of these descriptions of past events is to show that every realization listed in this book has been earned through actual experience, facing genuine challenges. As with other insights attained by other persons, once they enter the collective psyche, they belong to all of us. Buddha, Lincoln, Gandhi, the Wright Brothers, and others have blazed new paths in our consciousness, and their discoveries are now a part of our shared heritage, accessible to everyone.

To satisfy the reader's natural curiosity, my nearly seven-year ordeal of undocumented existence in New York came to an end when I met and married a beautiful lady.

CHAPTER THREE

Inception of the Insight

In 1992 I lived in New York City's East Village and regularly ran six to ten miles a couple times a week. I found these jogs to be the best meditation sessions. The body is engaged in a routine and familiar activity: The lungs are pumping, the legs are kicking—so the mind is free to visit beautiful places. I've always gotten the brightest ideas on these meditation runs. From my apartment on the corner of 9th Street and Avenue A, I'd run to East River Park, across the 10th Street overpass, and then along the water to the South Street Seaport and back. After the Williamsburg Bridge the path winds gently away from the river into the park, but when it comes back out to the water's edge, you get a clear view of Lower Manhattan and New York Harbor. And there, in her distant glory, stands the Statue of Liberty. She and I would have a rendezvous several times a week.

Insight = looking inside.

On one of these beautiful runs, of physical freedom and excursions of the mind, an insight emerged, somewhere from the crossings of the subconscious and the infinite. A number appeared: 102 years. Frankly, I didn't pay much attention to this at the time. I finished the run and went about my business, but the following day this thought was still there, and the following week, and the following month. This is when I got worried.

What was I going to do with this strange notion? What did it mean? Was this some kind of joke? Where did it come from, and what was I supposed to do with it?

Dear Albert, you once said, "There comes a time when the mind takes a higher plane of knowledge but can never prove how it got there."

Resistance and Doubts

Today I can simply say that I've had the notion that I'd live to be 102 since 1992, and the longer I live, the more I believe it. From this perspective it is also clear that it was absolutely necessary for me to pass through the darkest doubts of this insight to emerge on the other side confident in this knowledge. How can I assuage other people's legitimate concerns regarding the validity of this perception if I haven't first answered these doubts for myself?

Don't mistake doubts for weakness; only fools have no doubts. And if you can answer your doubts, you can strengthen your faith.

But it sure wasn't fun. Every initial suspicion, disbelief, and wonder that you may feel reading about this strange notion, I have experienced profoundly over the past twenty-six years in my body, heart, mind and in my daily life. For the first several years I fought and struggled with the idea, suspected it, didn't know what to make of it, was scared of it, mistrusted it, and tried to oppose it—but as it wouldn't go away I gradually yielded to it, researched it, understood it, accepted it, and finally came to rely on it. But let's take this development one step at a time.

I felt I couldn't tell anyone about this. They would laugh at me, or they would think I was hallucinating, that I thought too much of myself, that I had a big ego, or this was the kind of goofy thought you have after one too many drinks. Was this some kind of a cosmic joke, to set me up for ridicule and derision?

And where does this notion fit in my life, anyway? Do I now not mind how I behave, what I eat, and how I treat my body because I think I can live to be 102? Do I think I'm someone special to whom accepted rules of science and medicine don't apply? Are these thoughts the product of my overstimulated imagination playing tricks on me? Even if it were possible, what am I going to do with this idea? Do I think I'm a prophet, shaman, or visionary? Am I a charlatan or a clown? Am I grasping for significance? Is this a fool's errand? Following these anxieties came the mother of them all: What if somebody shoots me? After all, stuff happens.

Dark, disgusting fears attempt to paralyze my spirit. But doubts are not the opposite of faith, they are a part of faith. How will I react to natural skepticism of other people if I haven't addressed these reservations for myself? I need to go through the thick of these uncertainties, delve into them, and answer each of them. I need to expose this idea to the sunlight of clear inspection and see if it shrinks, dries, or shrivels. I need to look each one of these fears in the eye and conquer it, because the dragon that you slay gives you its power. This is how I grow stronger and smarter, and come to understand myself on a deeper level.

You have a heart as big as the world, but is this childish faith?

This question implies that would be juvenile, immature.

But if not this childish faith, then what?

No one just like you has ever walked the earth, felt what you feel, looked as you do.

You are by simple fact a unique specimen. When you are on your deathbed ready to cross over, will you look back on your entire journey and think I was not brave enough to trust in my creator?

Will you not travel the entire distance God assigned you?

Will you not accept the privilege and the responsibility for this vision?

If God says you can, are you going to convince yourself you can't?

What else will you regret not having done when you are ready to depart?

This period lasted several years, battling, brewing, and conflicting. But you go about your life, and you come to have faith. You try not to lose your sense of wonder, that private quiet instinct that says, "Why the heck not?" Is it frightening? I've dealt with darker thoughts. I've almost killed and have almost been killed. I am not afraid of this. And moreover, one day the bottom fell out from under that fear of being shot at random.

A new articulation surfaced and it made perfect sense; everything fell into place: If I am not killed prematurely, I'll live to be 102.

That is, within the domain over which I have control—my own behavior—I think that I can sustain life in this body for that long. Beyond this I have no control, and whatever happens is the will of the universe.

The four episodes, of almost dying and almost causing the death of others, made me realize that I don't have time to waste—not a day, not a moment. Life is too precious. I must do the most significant thing I conceive.

Acceptance and Beginning of Research

The idea would not leave my mind, so slowly and tentatively I began to examine it from different angles (let's see what happens; let the galaxies align in their proper positions). I continued to live my life, increasingly from the perspective of "If it were to happen, what would it mean in factual terms?": What would I have to think? How would I have to conduct myself? How would I have to breathe? Exercise? Eat? And what about what not to eat? (I have never denied myself of any kind of food; I enjoy everything in right proportions.)

As I gradually began to unravel the mystery of this strange notion, I recognized that this required of me a leap of faith—more than a leap, a full commitment. Because I'm a practical man who needs to feel the solid ground under my feet at all times, this was going to be a challenge. It was also clear that this curious calling was coming from a different place inside than the shallow, needy identity of an actor. I was hearing deeper truths, voices that were more profound and more substantive than I'd ever heard before. This new authority was located at the center of my being.

I am now entering new territories. New vistas are opening inside and out. I've never seen this idea so clearly: 102 years is the scaffolding God put on my life to prevent me from desperate actions. I won't do anything harmful to life. No short-cuts, no frenzy. God doesn't want me to break my neck. To last for this duration, I must stay healthy in body and mind.

Do I have the discipline to sustain myself through tedious days like today, dealing with the mind-numbing drudgery of existence? That old dread—that I'd wake up at eighty-five, look back on my life and say, "What the heck have I done?"—won't happen, because it's impossible to suddenly wake up at eighty-five if I haven't been sleeping all along. So keep examining your life. Keep asking yourself the tough questions of why you do what you do. But also be sure to have fun. The wisdom of the ages is distilled into this moment: Go fix yourself a bowl of fruit.

Buddha: "This is the secret of existence. Have faith in yourself, in the world, and in the fact that if you keep doing the right things while listening to your own rhythm, you're doing fine. You don't have to achieve anything. You don't have to get anywhere. This moment right here, one breath at a time, is your destination. You've arrived."

Reflect on revelation. Where do these insights come from? We don't get to choose our epiphanies. We don't wake up one day and say, "Today I'll have a brilliant idea about life!" By their nature, these notions originate in the Infinite Mind and lodge themselves in our psyche at a particular moment in time.

I instinctively understood that it was no accident why this insight appeared *now,* and not 1,000 years before or 1,000 years hence. We could not go to the moon before Orville and Wilbur Wright flew for the first time, as the scientific discoveries of the future will stand on the foundations of our present findings. We are a link in the chain of evolution, of our species, of knowledge, of universal consciousness.

My inner world had to catch up and gradually adjust to what my mind was discovering: that it is *possible.* I had to allow this new capacity into my psyche, and have faith that if I kept my feet firmly on the ground, which meant the most basic things (sleep well, eat well, treat yourself well, and treat those around you with the same decency you would like to be afforded to you) that this possibility might come true.

God, grant me the strength to serve this vision,
And guide me with plans to communicate it to others.

I couldn't resist these forces. If I did, I'd be at a conflict with myself, out of sync between my mind, heart, and body. This idea was pulling me in two distinct directions:

1. Research into health, longevity, nutrition, evolution, and psychology.
2. Incorporating the insights I was gaining into my body and in my everyday life.

I had to create harmony between the world at large and the world inside me. I had to regulate my energy, metabolism, behavior, and personal ambitions to fit the newly revealing structure in my life. An image of a framework of the length of time I might exist in this world was forming. I was beginning to see my body as a vessel into which a certain amount of fuel (energy) was poured, and it was my responsibility and privilege to decide how to use it. This was a new way of looking at existence—existence in general, and also my own: how to approach life; how to think of the past, present, and future; how to see myself in the larger context of the universe.

Here are some practical realizations that were emerging during this period and congealing into a coherent framework that I was beginning to see in my life:

Faith is an essential component in acquiring this new skill, but this faith is based on clear understanding of oneself and of how the world operates.

Do I know that this will happen? No. The nature of "knowing" is that we can't know what hasn't happened yet. But if it were to happen, this is how it would: through what we think and how we act.

If it's something good, and I can do it, then I *should* do it.

I was given this awareness not to show the world how smart and special I am but to first prove its validity in my life, and then teach it to others so they can use this power to improve their own lives.

It is the quality, not the quantity, of life that counts.

Due to advances in food production and distribution, as well as in medical treatments for advanced-age diseases, human life expectancy is increasing. The longest verified human life on record is 122 years and 164 days.[1] Even without accounting for the anticipated increase in human life span, within these known boundaries, any reasonable number we can conceive in accordance with our physical, mental, spiritual, and emotional states is valid.

The instinct to exist for that long is the life force in me—primal, eternal, the WILL to live: pulsing, driving, throbbing. My job is to harness and master it.

As I am a vessel, there are different liquids flowing through me, affecting my moods, digestion, energy levels, and overall health. My responsibility is to balance them.

Would I want to live forever? No, that would be tedious and pointless. Life is valuable because it is finite.

If I think that I know how long I could live, how does this account for illnesses and diseases? The correct way to think about this is that it is not a guarantee, a signed certificate that someone hands me saying, "You are promised to live 102 years." Rather, this is a *potential* that might come true if I make certain choices.

Regarding illnesses, it's not that healthy people don't get sick. But when they do, because they're healthy, they're able to fight off diseases more efficiently and to bounce back into full health more quickly. This also implies a personal responsibility on my part to keep myself in superb condition so I can prevent diseases from coming on.

I'd have to discover each day something worthy for which to live—finding meaning in the mundane.

On my larger journey of existence, this is where I am at present: Pace yourself.

It would only happen if I learn how to maintain superb physical, mental, and emotional conditions at every point of this journey—if I arrange my life so I can be the best version of myself at every stage.

I will have to strike a perfect balance between the childlike aspects of my psyche (trusting, boundless, imaginative, and innocent) and the mature man in me (pragmatic, prudent, competent, and responsible for my thoughts and actions).

Our power lies in understanding that the freedom and responsibility for our overall wellness are in our hands.

The future is open. We don't have to carry forward bad habits only because we've done them in the past.

We strive for certainties, but are obliged to operate within the structure of educated risks and prudent hopes. All life consists of making the best choices with less than perfect data. However, we know the basics: It's better not to smoke, it's better not to be overweight, it's better not to have addictions, it's better to stay physically and mentally active.

Therefore, out of the big void of uncertainty, I carve for myself a framework of consciousness: *This is how long I can exist in this world, and I support this decision with everyday choices.*

This meant arranging the mental furniture in my mind in such a way that living is fun and that I don't allow myself to sink into depression, darkness, negativity, or despair.

This new way of looking at life is my special gift to myself, a higher license and a challenge to sustain the potential life that I feel in my body for that long.

This is a confluence of art and science. There is a reason why this insight came to me and not someone else, at this time and no other, and at this particular place. It's because I've been doing the ring muscles daily since 1982. (We will go into ring muscles in detail later in the book.) They helped me to develop a deeper awareness of my physical being, which led to discovering dormant capacities in the body.

Granted, we don't know many things about the universe yet, but let this fact not paralyze us from acting on what we do know: the wisdom of our body, intuition, and health.

This is only a theory. I have to bear it out. If I am to do this, my number-one job is to live this potential out. This means that I'll be smart enough to do the simplest things right: Repeat my mantra of *eat well, sleep well, treat yourself and others well.* This whole premise rests on my ability to verify this hypothesis: I am test subject number one.

My contract with my creator is to realize the potential it has shown me. Just like emergency instructions on an airplane direct you to apply your oxygen mask first (before you attend to your loved ones), I'll never be able to help others if I don't first take good care of myself.

Ride this tiger gently. This is an enormous power; don't let it overwhelm you.

To master this tiger, I need to tap into my inner wisdom, and from that knowing perspective handle my passage through life.

Here's the clear elegance of it: My primary task is to live out this duration of 102. I can't do that if I worry myself to death. Everything I do has to resonate with this vision and has to fit in the overall framework this insight brings to my life.

This is how much time is allotted to me on earth.

Understanding how long I can live emphasizes the precarious and precious nature of existence.

This is also the solid ground on which I can stand and a license that is singularly my own. It is independent of anyone else. This I do when I'm totally on my own.

Melding faith and fact, it won't be possible without the underlying faith I have in this vision. However, that faith is implemented by hard, practical facts of good nutrition, an active lifestyle, proper rest, and life-work balance.

My primary goal, and the metric by which I'll be judged, is not to accomplish this deed or that, but to actually live out this duration that my creator has shown me.

From this perspective, the focus is health rather than accomplishing this deed or that.

How do I position myself physically and mentally so my behavior doesn't sacrifice my health?

This means a shift in priorities: Rather than struggling to meet the next goal and in the pursuit of that running myself down or making myself sick, my motivation becomes to maintain balance both in mind and body every step of the way.

It's not about me. I am serving this idea.

This is a critical point: If I can sense this, others can do it as well. I am not special, nor do I have extraordinary powers. This insight occurred to me, and I had the curiosity and character to investigate and understand it.

What is the biggest contribution I can make in life? That is my mission. Let me have faith to give voice to the best parts of me.

I need to own this vision. I need to accept the authority and responsibility for it. On this topic I know more than anyone else. On this I am the expert. I have to understand it and explain it to others clearly, methodically, and logically.

As I proceeded with this research over the years, it became evident that every new knowledge on the nature of existence that I gained had to be assimilated across three realms: first in my mind, then in my body, and finally tested in daily life. As the horizon was widening in my external world, my inner world was growing richer at the same time. My grip on life was strengthening, my freedom to think outside of preconceived notions was growing, and this process was allowing me to increasingly recognize and trust the internal processes of my body.

Buddha: Know thyself.

Alexander: You can.

Darwin: Use your wisdom.

Lincoln: How does it benefit others?

Einstein: Trust your imagination.

Mandela: Keep your eyes on the prize.

PART TWO

Scientific and Spiritual Foundations

We will now transition to exploring the scientific and spiritual foundations of our ability to sense how long we can live, and later the practical daily applications of this awareness that help us to live our longest and healthiest lives.

We are living at a remarkable period in time. The last one hundred years have given us more scientific discoveries than the entire preceding human history before them. We are the first generation to know the geometry, material composition, and evolution of the universe. Technological advances of long-distance telescopes such as Hubble and Planck have enabled us to see deeper into the cosmos than was previously possible and get a clear picture of the position of galaxies in space and time.

Emerging fields of new cosmology, neuroplasticity, superstring theory, and epigenetics are presenting a view of humankind as the eyes, ears, and mind of the cosmos with far more to discover in the world inside us than in the universe at large.

CHAPTER FOUR

New Cosmology and Superstring Theory

On September 25, 2012, the National Aeronautics and Space Administration (NASA) released a photo that shows the farthest view of the universe ever seen. The photo, called XDF for eXtreme Deep Field, was taken by the Hubble Space Telescope, and it goes back 13.2 billion years into the universe's past. The universe, in current scientific understanding, is thought to be 13.72 billion years old.

New cosmology aims to explain the nature of existence and the origins of life by presenting the universe as clearly as possible. The consensus in the scientific community regarding the chronology of the cosmos is as follows:

Evolution of the Universe (approximate numbers)

13.72 billion years ago: What we call "the big bang" occurs, resulting in the release of matter and energy. We don't currently know for certain what preceded the big bang, but there are several theories, such as serial universes (existing one after the other,) multiple dimensions (which we cannot detect at present,) or many universes existing at once—a multiverse. There's also a theory that the universe emerged from nothingness, which we will discuss later in the book

4.54 billion years ago: The Earth forms from the stellar ash that had been released during the big bang. We humans are made of the same ingredients as the planets and stars. Every atom in our body comes from planet Earth, which in turn is made of the same energy and matter as everything else in the cosmos.

3.5 billion years ago: The first living microbes appear on Earth.

2.4 billion years ago: Plant and animal life are plentiful on Earth.

300 million years ago: Our ancestors diverge from bird species and come down from trees.

200 million years ago: Mammals arise.

65 million years ago: Primates emerge.

7 million years ago: Homo hominids (man-like) break away from the other hominids (great apes: gorillas, gibbons, orangutans, chimpanzees); bipedalism evolves.

400,000 years ago: The controlled use of fire by upright walking hominids (Homo erectus) is common. This was a significant developmental threshold, because it meant mastery of the environment and ability to migrate and inhabit areas that previously were inhospitable to life.

300,000 years ago: Anatomically modern humans (Homo sapiens sapiens) emerge.

50,000 years ago: Behaviorally modern humans arise.

1543 CE: Nicolaus Copernicus publishes *On the Revolutions of the Celestial Spheres,* which introduces the awareness that Earth is not at the center of the universe, but revolves around the sun, and triggers the Scientific Revolution and the Enlightenment.

In order to grasp the extent of the universe, let's consider a few key facts that define it. As of writing this chapter (October 2017), this is what our latest science knows about the cosmos we inhabit. To make things as simple as possible (but not any simpler, to follow the sage advice of Einstein), let's use here the metaphor of peeling layers of an onion, from the outermost layer of the universe that we know we will travel increasingly closer to planet Earth.

We currently don't know how much of the universe there actually is. The most advanced instruments available can't tell us the boundaries of the cosmos. The slice of space and time that we can see today is 90 billion light years across, but we know that beyond there is more space, and we know that this space is expanding. It's been known for almost a century that the universe is expanding and has been doing so since right after the big bang. The universe today is nearly 1,000,000,000,000 (1 trillion) times larger than it was when it was just one second old, right after the explosion of the big bang.[1]

Ninety-five percent of the universe is invisible to us because it's made of what we currently call "dark energy" and "dark matter." Obviously, putting these labels on those forces is a sign of our current ignorance of their true nature. These are temporary designations until our measurements and observations will be able to explain them clearly. We are doing now what we've always done as conscious and curious beings: pushing the boundaries of the darkness that surrounds us. We can easily imagine our early ancestors roughly 400,000 years ago lighting the recently tamed fire after darkness fell to illuminate their immediate area in the open field, to ward off predators and feel safer and in better control of their environment. As an inherent trait, and for the long-term survival of our species, we are following today the same instinct.

Dark energy can be described as the opposite of gravity. Gravity pulls things together, whereas dark energy pushes them apart. Dark energy is a relatively new concept (discovered in 1999), and it causes the universe to accelerate its expansion. Most recent observations indicate that dark energy accounts for approximately 69 percent of the universe.[2]

Physicists consider the origin and nature of dark energy as the biggest mystery facing their field at present. Cosmologists and physicists have no idea how dark energy originates, the assumption being that it is somehow related to the origin of the universe.[3] This fact illustrates once again that although we have come a long way in understanding ourselves and the universe, we still have a very long way to go. Although to our predecessors from 10,000 and 1,000 years ago we might seem advanced and sophisticated, to humans living 1,000 and 10,000 years from now, this period in our evolution will look like an infant making its first steps in the world.

Dark matter comprises roughly 26 percent of the universe.[4] Dark matter is not made of atoms and molecules like we are, because atoms and molecules absorb, emit, and interact with light, but not *this* dark matter. Its gravitational pull is responsible for the position of galaxies in the cosmos.

The remainder of the known cosmos, ordinary matter made of atoms—the stuff that makes up stars, galaxies, planets, and everything visible—accounts for a relatively tiny 5 percent of the universe.[5]

In October 2016 new data collected from Hubble Space Telescope revealed that there are at least 10 times more galaxies in the observable universe than astronomers previously thought, raising the earlier estimate of 200 billion galaxies to the current count of 2 trillion. This discovery of formerly unknown galaxies means that 90 percent of the known galaxies in the universe have yet to be studied.[6]

The average distance between each galaxy is roughly 3 million light years. Light travels at the speed of 186,000 miles per second. Speed of light is considered the speed limit in the cosmos.[7]

Galaxies are moving away from each other at an accelerating speed, which leads to the conclusion that because galaxies in the future will be receding away from us at faster-than-light speed, this will make them invisible to us.[8] Because their speed of recession from us will be greater than the speed at which light travels, they will have broken through that speed barrier and will have disappeared from our horizon. This again shows that we are living in a dynamic, ever-changing universe in which we—our minds, bodies, energies—are in a constant flux. What we are today is different than what we were yesterday. As we'll detail further in Chapter 9, in a year you recycle 98 percent of matter in your body.[9]

Tomorrow, and next year, and twenty years from now, you will be the person you are today, but in a whole new configuration.

The big bang counts as the beginning of the universe as we understand it today. Cosmologists were able to determine that the big bang happened 13.72 billion years ago because of cosmic microwave background radiation (CMBR). The CMBR is the afterglow of the light and energy released at the big bang. As our high-powered telescopes enable us to see further and further into the cosmos, this means earlier and earlier in its existence, because, as we mentioned, distance in the universe is measured in light years. When we see more distant galaxies and stars we are going back in time, because it takes that much longer for that light to reach us—millions of light years.

To add another astounding fact to this discussion, recent studies find three times as many stars in the universe as previously thought. The new approximate number of stars is 1 with 23 zeroes.

What was there before the big bang? The best scientific answer available today is that there was a potential for space, time, energy, matter, and everything that would happen in the future. Of course, because we have not yet reached the end of time, that journey of evolution and discovery of the possibilities that end up being observable phenomena will continue as long as we live. If human consciousness in the universe no longer exists, it begs the philosophical question of whether any kind of awareness will remain—as in the old conundrum of, if a tree fell in the forest and there was nothing there to record it, how can we be certain that it made any sound?

The big bang was an eruption of energy and light that occurred everywhere at once. Humankind is the furthest advanced life form to evolve from the forces unleashed at the big bang. The human brain is the most complex computational machine currently known to exist in the universe, and the human mind is the primary known conveyor of consciousness in the cosmos.

We are the offspring of supernovas. We are made of star dust. The carbon, oxygen, nitrogen, and iron in our body could not be created in the universe in any other way than through the collapse and explosion of a star. Also, it's very likely that the atoms in your leg came from a different star than the atoms in your hand. Our bodies are celestial bodies made of the same stuff of which the planets and stars are made.

Stars go through the cycle of birth and death to allow the birth of humans. We are a further incarnation of a star. We are embedded in this evolutionary process: Just as a single drop in an ocean contains in it the character of the entire ocean, so each of us carries in our genes the entire information of existence. In our cells, everything exists as a potential.

The echoes of these distant events live in our body—in our genetic makeup and in our bloodstream. The universe exists in each of us. The cosmos wants to come to self-awareness and humankind serves as its eyes, ears, mental processors, communication means, and instruments of further evolution.

To illustrate the intricacy of the universe that produced the human species, consider that the sun is ninety-three million miles away from Earth. If it was two feet closer we would burn up, and if it was two feet further we would freeze. We are a product of this delicate, intelligent cosmic balance, and whether a person attributes this to the hand of God, science, self-organizing principles, spirit, or the unified field of consciousness, it is impossible to discount the creative organizing intelligence that made all this possible.

Consciousness in the universe has been unfolding for the past 13.7 billion years since the big bang. We humans, the most advanced conduit of consciousness in the cosmos, are at the present stage of evolution, and have not reached our final form. The perception of our duration is a natural step in our future progress.

To quote physical chemist Lothar Schafer, "Evolution is not a process of adapting bodies to the environment, but of adapting our minds to increasingly complex forms in the cosmic potentiality. Evolution is a development of mind, not of bodies."[10]

So what are we as humans? The most developed link in the cosmic chain of evolution. Our ancestors are our individual family predecessors, and earlier than that a common human ancestor, and earlier still an animal ancestor, and a microbial ancestor, all the way back to the eruption of the big bang. We carry in our cells 13.7 billion years of information, and also all the possible scenarios of the future.

From this perspective, what is existence? It is awareness; the state of being sentient; an ongoing quest for knowledge. We humans are at the frontiers of evolution, moving the universe forward with our thoughts and actions.

Just as Copernicus shattered the worldview that existed nearly five centuries ago of Earth as the center of the universe, so today we are faced with rapidly shifting mental plates on the nature of existence. If we stop this process of exploration we will atrophy and die. But this really is a phantom fear, because, being what we are, we can't stop probing. We are built this way. It is in our genes to investigate and go further than where we were yesterday. If we accept it, our designated role in this elaborate framework is to awaken the cosmos to higher consciousness.

Let's do a little exercise.

General Note: For the exercises listed in this book, first read each one aloud as you record your voice, and then play them back. This way, you don't need to hold the book to follow the instructions.

Remember those evolutionary markers earlier in this chapter of first primates, mammals, and living organisms coming into existence? Let's go back in time to the big bang. Get comfortable in your chair and concentrate on your breath. Breath is the main doorway to enter your inner world. Breathe in, breathe out, breathe in, breathe out. Establish a steady, deep, and effortless rhythm of breaths.

Now think of the oldest relative in your family—the earliest ancestor that you're aware of, even if they passed on before you were born. Think of them clearly for five seconds.

Okay, now let's go further back to our common human ancestor. Let's visit a tribe of cavemen and cavewomen sitting by the fire. Let's stay here for five seconds. Look around you with your mind's eye. See the field where you're sitting, and notice if it's cold or warm, if it's day or night.

Now let's go further back to a single-cell amoeba, and from there jump back to when planet Earth came into existence from the stellar debris that was floating in space roughly 4.54 billion years ago.

And now let's jump all the way back to the eruption of the big bang— a grand explosion of light and energy occurring everywhere at once. Let's stay in this mental place for five seconds.

Now gradually we'll start coming back to the present. Let's go to planet Earth forming, and skip to first living microbes, to the cavemen and women, and slowly back into the present moment. Make sure you're breathing steady and free. Get comfortable in your seat and let's continue.

We just visited 13.7 billion years of evolution. This is the past that we carry in our genes. You are a result of this entire history. As Carl Sagan noted, if you want to make an apple pie from scratch you have to start at the big bang.

Looking forward, because we have not yet reached the end of time, we have not yet reached the end of our potential. We simply don't know what it is because existence means constant change, mutation, progress. As we discover more about the universe at large we understand more about the world inside us, and vice versa, in a mutually dependent evolution of scientific and spiritual awareness.

As we will discuss in detail further along these pages, the worlds within and without are interconnected and interdependent. We humans are not a foreign entity that was randomly inserted into this universe from outside. We are made of similar building blocks of energy and matter of which the planets and stars are made.

Every atom in our body comes from planet Earth, which in turn is made of the components of the galactic ash, which resulted from the explosion of the big bang. We are part of this ever-changing, dynamic continuum, and we are linking in our present form those distant pasts and futures. The path on which we walk unfolds as we advance.

We move through space with the other celestial bodies, and the same energy that animates them also animates us. Until we find otherwise, we are the most advanced intelligence existing in the world.

Superstring Theory

As we saw earlier, the most accurate estimates that our space instruments provide show that roughly 69 percent of the knowable universe is what cosmologists call "dark energy," a mysterious force that defies gravity and is responsible for speeding up the universe's rate of expansion. Approximately 26 percent of the universe is dark matter, which does not interact with light. The basic unit of matter is atoms, but what this dark matter is made of we don't yet know. We know this is not Earth matter or star matter, it is something completely new that science still hasn't determined.[11] And about 5 percent is the visible universe, ordinary matter made of atoms: stars, galaxies, and planets.

Within this premise, modern physics has tried to devise a single unified theory that would explain the nature of the universe while accounting for all its moving parts. Isaac Newton formulated the principles of universal gravitation roughly three centuries ago. The theory of relativity, which Einstein developed at the beginning of the twentieth century, deals with the macro level of planets, galaxies, and the larger cosmos.

Quantum theory, developed by (the telescope's namesake) Max Planck and colleagues concurrently with and slightly after the theory of relativity, studies the micro realm of atomic and subatomic planes. And superstring theory, which follows quantum mechanics, is a theoretical framework that has been developing for the past thirty years that aims to understand the fundamental structure of the universe. Of course, every scientific theory builds on those that came before it, so it is a bit arbitrary to mark the birth of superstring theory in the 1980s, but that is the beginning of when this theory started to be studied and debated in earnest.

Superstring theory gives us this understanding of existence:

- Everything is made of particles.
- Particles contain atoms and molecules.
- Molecules contain two or more atoms.
- Atoms contain protons, neutrons, and electrons.

- Protons and neutrons contain quarks.
- Quarks contain no more matter but strings of vibration—
  pure energy.

From Newtonian particle physics of hard, tangible objects we move down into the atomic level, then sub-atomic, then nuclear, and then sub-nuclear. When we divide the particles down to their tiniest ingredients to discover what they're made of, what we're left with is strings of probabilities, vibrations of potential. Matter forms out of formlessness—out of abstraction. We discover that there is nothing more to touch, or to hold, that life in its essence is pure energy and information. This is the source of you and the cosmos.

Quantum theory shows us that at the level of what is called the Planck Scale, which is ten million-million-million times smaller than the atomic nucleus, consciousness is the foundation of the universe. It is the source of energy, information, space, time, and matter. In this unified field of consciousness, everything exists as a potential. Because we are made of the same building blocks as the stars and the planets, the consciousness that informs the universe also informs our bodies.

Quantum mechanics present particles as units of energy (*quantum* means unit) with wave-like properties, which adjust their behavior according to who is observing them and what experiment is being conducted. Quantum mechanics show that an individual's thoughts actually trigger the reaction of matter at the quantum level. The expectations of the experimenter cause the experiment's outcome. This means that we have a definite influence on the world around us. Our thoughts affect the physical world in which we live. At the quantum level, our subjective awareness locks an objective reality into position.

Any potential is just a probability until you or I freeze it into reality—fix it into existence through observation and application. Particles begin as pure potential that vibrates as strings of probabilities, and they collapse into being an actual particle only when we direct our attention on them. When reality is locked into position by awareness, it cannot shift.

When something is not observed by awareness, it exists in a formless state of potential.

Let's use here again the image of peeling the onion of existence. Each layer that we peel gets us closer to our essence. And when we strip these layers of existence and reach down to our core as far as our current science allows, down to this unified field, we discover that at our source we, and the universe, are nothing but pure energy, pure potential waiting to be realized—according to the laws of nature.

At this unified field, we humans are the perfect embodiment of the cosmos, because we are made of the building blocks of the universe. The human body is a small autonomous planet informed with cosmic energy and intelligence. As Michio Kaku, professor of theoretical physics at the City College of New York and CUNY Graduate Center, says, "A human body can think thoughts, play a piano, kill germs, remove toxins, make a baby all at once. Once it's doing that your biological rhythms are actually mirroring the symphony of the universe."[12]

Every thought, emotion, sensation, and feeling in our body is made of energy. Each thought has a distinctive electrical signature of its own, and is a potent, dynamic force with enormous power. There is no reality in the absence of observation, and observation creates reality. This means that you as the observer create the subjective reality you are observing.

In this unified field where everything is possible, anything that would improve our lives is desirable. In this book we ask ourselves: What good is it to know how long I could live? The simple answer is that this knowledge gives us self-awareness and enables us to go through life with full command of our inner resources.

To bridge this moment between the past and future, let's recall Buddha's quote from 2,600 years ago: "The mind is everything. What you think you become."

One of the basic principles of what is called "quantum weirdness" is that anything that is not forbidden by the fundamental laws of nature, can and will happen. Anything that can happen, will eventually happen. Our capacity to sense how long we can live currently exists in a formless state of probabilities among infinite other probabilities in the universe and in our genes. We freeze it into reality—isolate it into existence—by directing our attention and intention on it.

This is what we are in our essence: a thought, an idea, a unit of energy; and we manifest those ideas in reality by the choices we make in our everyday lives.

CHAPTER FIVE

Neuroplasticity and Epigenetics

et's begin this chapter also by presenting a wider view of what neuro-science currently knows about the brain as related to our subject and then gradually move into a tighter focus on our topic.

Scientists have learned more about the human brain in the past ten years than in all other time periods combined. Our brains contain eighty-six to one hundred billion neurons, or nerve cells, which have trillions of connections, or synapses. Each neuron is connected to up to 10,000 other neurons, which means that the number of synapses in our brain is between one hundred trillion and one quadrillion.[1]

Signals between neurons in our brains are carried by chemicals called "neurotransmitters." With the trillions of connections firing constantly to intake and process information, neuroscience today simply doesn't know the limits of what the brain is capable of.[2] To emphasize the point made previously on these pages, we have not reached the end of understanding of ourselves and the world.

Neuroplasticity is the ability of the brain to constantly adapt to changing circumstances throughout life. *Neuro* refers to *neuron*, the cells in our brains and nervous systems. *Plasticity* refers to *plastic*: flexible and changeable. Neuroplasticity enables the brain to regularly form new communication pathways between these cells and continuously reconfigure existing ones. This process enables us to acquire different skills, memorize new information, and generally adapt to existence through experience.

The prevailing agreement in mainstream medicine used to be that brain development was largely complete by the end of childhood. Neuroscientists believed that the process of neural regeneration (forming new cells and creating new connections) stopped, and that brain structure was fixed and "hardwired" by this time. However, research since the beginning of the twenty-first century has shown that the brain's neural connections never reach a fixed pattern that cannot change further. Rather, recent studies are showing that the brain is changing constantly, in response to learning, disease, exercise, and other stimuli, through our entire life span. This process is called "neurogenesis": the brain produces new neurons until the day we die.

This freshly understood innate plasticity of the human brain across the length of a lifetime carries with it enormous implications in personal, social, medical, and developmental fields. In practical terms relevant to our topic, this means that a person can stay active and engaged in life for as long as they practice a lifestyle that stimulates both the body and the mind.

Because of the insights of neuroscience, recently there has been an explosion of understanding about how the brain is involved in every aspect of health. Take a moment to consider this: If the brain can change itself, that means that how we think about everything in life can change as well. You can change how you view your diet, health, relationships, and how you think about yourself and your place in the world. In short, as you get to know yourself and the universe better, you can apply these new understandings to improve your life. Tomorrow is not yesterday. Your entire future is ahead of you, open, unwritten, malleable, ready for you to do with it what you wish.

With every thought and feeling we reshape the neural networks in our brains. The higher quality of our thoughts, the better lives we create. If you look at it correctly, the best years of your life can be ahead of you.

Your body changes and it cannot do at forty-five what it did at eighteen. However, your understanding of yourself has now grown, you don't need to repeat past mistakes, and you can make choices that balance all the aspects of your mind, body, and spirit.

Neuroplasticity is a vast and promising field that is revealing extraordinary possibilities both on an individual level and on the level of our entire species. For example, new studies show that the brain is able to reorganize itself in response to unforeseen circumstances and traumas. One remarkable illustration of this is sensory substitution, in which in a person who had lost their sight, an area in the brain dedicated to processing vision, is now drafted to processing enhanced hearing and touch.

Moreover, other organs in your body can start to function in brand new ways, such as seeing through your tongue. This might seem to make no sense, but as David Eagleman, adjunct professor at the department of psychiatry and behavioral sciences at Stanford University, writes in his 2015 book, *The Brain: The Story of You*, "Keep in mind that seeing is never anything but electrical signals streaming into the darkness of your skull. Normally this happens via the optic nerves, but there is no reason the information can't stream in via other nerves instead. As sensory substitution demonstrates, the brain takes whatever data comes in and figures out what it can make of it."[3]

I am including the publication years of the books cited on these pages in the Notes section of this book, so the reader can appreciate the rapid rate of discoveries we are experiencing constantly about our inner and outer worlds.

Another recently revealed feature of neuroplasticity is that the brain changes its structure as we think.[4] The quality of our thoughts determines the quality of our brains, and in a larger sense, the quality of our lives. In a self-perpetuating loop, what we think and how we behave creates certain outcomes; those results in return affect our reactions to them and thus the structure of our brain. As we will see later, our brains are energy fields that send out particle waves in the form of thought and expectation. Although accidents and random events do happen, in large part we create the outcomes that we anticipate. This is why it is critical to be mindful of the ways we think about ourselves and the world, because if we see bad things and expect bad things, bad things are liable to happen. Conversely, if our intentions are life-affirming and positive, and we support our actions with foresight, patience, wisdom, and conscientiousness, our world and the place we inhabit in it is affected accordingly.

From the perspective of humankind as the eyes and mind of the cosmos, neuroplasticity plays an essential part in the universe's ability to adapt, evolve, and deepen its self-awareness through the human species.

Buddha: *Know thyself.*

Alexander: *You can.*

Darwin: *Be smart.*

Lincoln: *How does it help others?*

Einstein: *Trust yourself.*

Mandela: *Be responsible.*

Body Postures

Sitting position is considered the most comfortable posture for mind-body exercises without inducing sleep.

Sitting position is a convenient way of doing meditative exercises because it can be used effortlessly at almost any location. You can use this position at home, on a short break at work, out in the park, in an airport, or even on a bus.

Lying position is an ideal posture in which to do deep meditative body work.

This position can be used for every exercise listed on these pages. If you find yourself falling asleep, and your schedule allows a nap, it is good, as this is a sign that your body requires rest. As we will discuss in Chapter 10, there are many health benefits to restorative sleep, during which the body regains its innate equilibrium. In a meditation session, if you find that you are falling asleep unintentionally, switch to the sitting position and continue your concentration in this posture. The final decision of what posture to use is yours. Listen to your body and choose the position in which you feel most relaxed and at ease.

In addition, it will benefit you to start considering your mind/body/energy as a single unit, with each part influencing the others and dependent on others for your overall wellness in life.

Exercise: Releasing Energy Blocks in Your Body

This practice is effective for generating free flow of energy and cleansing toxins from your body. It can be used separately for these purposes, and it can also be combined with a relaxation routine.

It is best to do this exercise in the lying position, with your legs stretched out on the floor to their full length. It's also recommended here to use earplugs, to shut out outside noise and draw into your inner peace. Allow at least 20 minutes for this sequence.

If you're currently dealing with a particular ailment, it is your responsibility to find out whether this condition requires medical attention, in which case you should get it without delay.

As a general instruction for doing this routine, if you see that you are running out of time before it's completed, it's better to stop in whichever area of your body you are, and next time simply resume the exercise where you'd left off. It is better to be thorough than rush the process.

Lie down comfortably at your favorite place, stretch your body on the floor, and follow your breath into your center.

Establish a free, easy, steady pattern of breaths.

Run a mental checklist of your limbs—how your arms, legs, neck, and abdomen feel.

Take stock of the different systems of your body: heartbeat, digestion, your current emotional state, and your overall physical feeling. Do you feel sluggish, stressed, tense, or anxious?

Notice what part of your body feels the best, and what part feels the least well. The goal of this exercise is to concentrate on this troubled area of your body to understand what causes this unease and solve it.

It is important to realize that the blockages discussed in this sequence are not obvious lumps that you can detect with your fingers (although in severe cases this can also be true) but are better thought of as "knots" of energy, in liquid and fluid terms. Your aim is to release this obstruction in your body by focusing your attention on it, so it can be washed into the blood stream and dissolve as salt in water.

This mental blockage can be the result of poor blood flow into this area. Energize this area by directing clean and warm focus into it, and prudently, without harming yourself, rub it gently with your fingers to melt and diffuse this knot in your body.

Make sure you don't create unintentional tightness in other parts of your body as you concentrate your attention on melting this knot.

Rest, breathe deeply, stretch to your full length, and listen to your body.

You might feel the need to readjust on the floor, or to move your limbs, which are signs that your body is realigning itself with a free flow of energy.

It is helpful to begin thinking of this process as taking place both in space and time. This means listening to and respecting your body's inner rhythms. Your body has its natural pace, and it cannot be rushed or shortened.

Now slowly bring this routine to an end. Make sure your breath is steady and effortless. Roll to your side, rise from the floor in an effortless manner, and rejoin your day.

Note: *Here and elsewhere in the book we will emphasize that you need to find your comfort zone—your sense of fun—as you do these exercises because it is your privilege and freedom to live a healthy and happy life. This is not something you will do for a short time, as some people take up a diet for six months, lose weight, think they'd accomplished their goal, get back to their old habits, and regain their weight. Your purpose here is to acquire simple and useful routines for a lifetime and apply them in your daily existence, which will make you feel vibrant, clean physically and mentally, and centered in your body and mind.*

Epigenetics

Dictionary definition:

Epi: above, beyond

Genetics: the makeup of an organism or group of organisms

Epigenetics is an emerging scientific field that goes beyond the old notion of "nature versus nurture" by showing that instead of pitting these two aspects against each other, over the course of a person's lifetime both these features play crucial roles in forming a full existence.

Epigenetics has been developing for the past few decades and is steadily becoming a central model in new biology. It demonstrates that contrary to long-held beliefs, DNA is not the determining element in a person's quality and quantity of life, but something that can be tinkered with and bent to our will. Our DNA serves as a blueprint to the life we build through our thoughts and actions.

Biologist Bruce Lipton, in his landmark 2006 book, *The Biology of Belief,* describes epigenetics as the "new science of self-empowerment." According to Lipton, "The notion that only physical molecules can impact cell physiology is outmoded. Biological behavior can be controlled by invisible forces, including thought, as well as it can be controlled by physical molecules like penicillin."[5]

It is no coincidence that the pattern we see in superstring theory of life at its essence, being a unit of pure potential influenced by outside forces, is similar to the principle of existence we see in biological cells where, as Lipton further writes, "The cell's operations are primarily molded by its interaction with the environment, not by its genetic code."[6]

This understanding that the environment is chiefly responsible for a cell's destiny directly relates to the point made earlier in this chapter that an individual can stay healthy in an old age by practicing a lifestyle (i.e., creating the environment) that *stimulates both the body and the mind.*

Epigenetics reveal that our consciousness modulates our biology. Our thoughts affect our genes and not the other way around. Genes carry our particular information, but they are not fixed and final. They're malleable, and are influenced by what we think, how we feel, and our environment.

Mind controls the body. Thoughts—new information—create new forms. Epigenetics puts the power to adjust your genetic blueprint in your own hands. Your thoughts and intentions are more conducive to health than drugs because energy is more potent in affecting matter than chemicals.

How does the mind influence the body? What is the biological mechanism by which this process takes place inside us? As Norman Doidge, professor at the University of Toronto's department of psychiatry, explains in his 2007 book, *The Brain that Changes Itself,* the genes we are born with play two distinct roles. One is the "template role," which refers to the genes' ability to replicate themselves and pass on information to the next generation of genes. This is a built-in process that is outside of our conscious control. The other is the "transcription role." Each of our cells contains all our genes. However, not all those genes are expressed, or turned on, all the time. When a gene is turned on, it makes a protein that changes the structure and operation of the cell. This transcription role is affected by what we think and what we do.[7] This is how the thoughts in our mind affect what happens in our body.

Recent medical studies show that the relationship between genes and lifestyle choices in determining the length and quality of our life is 30 to 70 percent in favor of lifestyle choices.[8] In other words, how we think of ourselves, the world, health, longevity, and our overall approach to life play the deciding role in the quality and quantity of our duration on earth.

As noted in Chapter 4, we live in a participatory universe. We manifest the outcome that we anticipate. Our brains are energy fields that send out particle waves in the form of thought and expectation. When we focus our attention on the number of years that we sense that we can reasonably live in this body, we cause the body to adjust itself to this new consciousness.

The fact that perception controls biology leads to the realization that the person most responsible for our overall wellness is ourselves. Here's the mental switch: You don't have to see yourself as declining in health as you age. Rather, you're making choices that would enable you to be the best version of yourself at every age. Instead of an unwitting instrument of the genetics you've inherited, you are the conscious master of your journey through life, determining your destiny by what you think and how you act.

Exercise: Ride Your Breath into Your Center

Breath is the easiest way to enter your inner world, to regroup, center, and balance yourself.

Allow at least twenty minutes for this exercise. Choose a comfortable environment (your preferred room, study, or another quiet part of your home). Set your favorite conditions in this room (curtains drawn or open, pleasant temperature, and so on). Wear loose clothes that will enable you to lie or sit without feeling tightness. Sweatpants and baggy clothes are perfect for this purpose.

At the beginning, it is recommended that you use earplugs because they will help you to shut out the outside world and direct your attention inward. They will also help you to reduce external noise so you can listen more freely to the rhythms and currents flowing in your body.

It's recommended to lie down for this exercise, but if you find that you're dozing off, switch to the sitting position.

Lie or sit down in a free, uncluttered place where you'll be able to roll around if you wish. Make yourself comfortable. Stretch and shake your limbs. Be sure that your head, neck, and shoulders are not tight. If they are, gently roll your head from left to right and back several times, always with a sense of ease, never with force, and never with pressure.

Shake your hands as you let out a sound (Hahh Hahh, Hahh, Hahh) to expel tension from your body. Do this for as long as it's pleasant, and until you feel ready inside to begin listening to your heartbeat and breath. Paying attention to your breath and heartbeat allows you to get in closest possible touch with your body and understand its natural rhythm.

As you lie or sit in your position, inhale and exhale deeply several times without trying to control anything. Simply let your body do what it does naturally as you monitor your breath.

Don't expect or anticipate any big revelations at this stage. Just listen to your heartbeat. The purpose of this routine is for you to begin developing awareness of the energy flow in your body. Your body is the vessel in which you live, your first and most important home.

Follow your breath and heartbeat in this manner for five minutes, as you do a mental checklist of how the different areas of your body feel (shoulders, chest, abdomen, thighs, knees, and so on).

Now think of the fact that your heartbeat and your breath are interconnected and interdependent in the same way that your body and mind are inseparable parts of your being.

Meditate on your breath with these questions:

- Is my breath shallow or deep?
- Is it fast or slow?
- Am I feeling any difficulty or displeasure while I breathe?
- Is my heart beating evenly or do I detect any syncopated rhythm?
- Can I feel the blood pumping into my heart?
- Is there tightness in my body?
- Do I feel tired or energetic?
- Do I feel sluggish or refreshed?
- Does my body feel light? Heavy? Fit? Soft?
- Do I feel impatient? Bothered?
- Can I enjoy myself lying in this position following my breath and heartbeat?

You don't need to pass judgment on any of these conditions, because the aim at present is for you to simply develop awareness of the processes taking place in your body.

Rest, let go, and gradually bring this exercise to an end. As you slowly get up, you will feel relaxed, centered, and refreshed.

This has been an important step in your gaining access to the internal processes of your body. Repeat this routine as many times as you desire. In its simple and effortless manner, it will be your doorway into your inner world. To begin future exercises, it's helpful to use this personal mantra: *Ride my breath into my center.*

As this fun exercise shows, you shouldn't expect spectacular overhead fireworks when you lie or sit down to these quiet routines. Rather, the practice you are doing is minute, private, reaches deep inside you, and evolves over time. These exercises are better thought of not as fireworks but as tapping the deposits of wisdom stored in your body, which have been passed down to you over generations to culminate in the perfect instrument of existence you are today. As you do these simple exercises regularly, your body will regain its original equilibrium, and you will begin to trust the messages your body is communicating to you on a consistent basis. The next step for you will be to create the circumstances in your life where your body and mind can be at their best condition, operating seamlessly to inform and strengthen each other.

CHAPTER SIX

Optimal Duration
of Existence

The biological foundation of our ability to sense how long we can live rests in the genetic fact that every living organism has an optimal duration of existence. This is the number of years that they are expected to live under ideal conditions. For example, shrews, who typically live two years, and whales, who on average live eighty, both have approximately one billion and a half heartbeats in a lifetime. (One whale species, the bowhead, can live up to 200 years, but this species is considered an outlier in terms of whale life expectancy.)

These two very different animals have the same amount of energy proportionate to their bodies, but they operate at different frequencies. The whale's heart beats in a low and steady rhythm at about six beats per minute (BPM)—one heartbeat every ten seconds—whereas the shrew's heart beats in a much faster pace, at approximately 600 BPM—ten heartbeats every one second. It burns up its energy a lot quicker.

In humans, as in animals, a fast heart rate means that the heart has to work harder. However, unlike wild creatures who are blind instruments of their DNA, we humans have the capacity to understand the amount of energy in our body and use this energy in the manner that we choose. Humans, on average, have two billion and a half heartbeats in a lifetime.

Optimal duration of existence refers to the maximum amount of years that a living organism can last under the most favorable circumstances. The following chart lists the life expectancies of various animal species.[1]

African Grey Parrot	73	Galapagos Land Tortoise	193
American Alligator	56	Goat	15
American Box Turtle	123	Greenland Shark	400
Angleworm	15	Hippopotamus	25
Ant—Queen	3	Horse	30
Ant—Worker	½	Koala	8
Bat	24	Lion	35
Bear	40	Mongoose	12
Beaver	20	Mouse	4
Bee—Queen	5	Ox	20
Bee—Worker	1	Platypus	10
Bowhead whale	200	Porcupine	20
Bull	28	Quail	7
Camel	50	Rabbit	9
Carp	100	Rattlesnake	22
Cat	25	Rhinoceros	40
Chicken	14	Sheep	15
Cow	22	Snapping Turtle	57
Deer	26	Tiger	22
Dog	22	Wolf	18
Donkey	45	Wombat	15
Elephant	70	Woodchuck	15
Fox	14	Wood Duck	22

The Greenland shark is considered the longest living vertebrate on the planet. Just as with human life spans, the actual lifetime of a specific animal may be significantly shorter than the optimal numbers listed in the chart when diet or environmental conditions are poor.

Human life expectancy around the world has been steadily increasing for the past 200 years. This has been mainly due to improvements in education, housing, and sanitation, leading to drops in early and midlife mortality, which were primarily caused by infections. Further developments of vaccines and antibiotics, and the recent declines in later-life mortality, have contributed to this trend of longer life expectancy that is currently increasing at a rate of approximately two years per decade.[2]

As we see, these improvements are mainly due to lifestyle changes, rather than to any genetic adaptations of our species. This is another perspective on the recent studies discussed earlier in the book that lifestyle choices play the predominant role in the length of a person's lifespan. It is no surprise that the advances in living standards caused by the shift to modern living conditions, and wider access to shelter, food, clothes, and medicine lead to lower mortality rates and result in rising life expectancies throughout the world. As a stark illustration, the rate of improvement in our life expectancy made only in the last century is greater than the improvement made during the entire history of evolution from chimpanzees to humans.

We are living longer in every country in the world. The current global life expectancy is around seventy-one years and about ninety years in Monaco, where, according to the CIA World Factbook page, people live longer than any other country. The longest verified human life on record belongs to the late Jeanne Louise Calment, who lived in France to the age of 122.4 years.

In the United States, life expectancy today is an average of seventy-nine years, and the continuing increase in longevity means that approximately 10,000 people turn sixty-five every day, and one in five Americans will be over sixty-five by 2030.[3]

Let's draw the distinction between longevity and life span. "Longevity" refers to the growing field of research that looks into extending the amount of years humans live. Longevity implies a lengthy life and is defined in humans as living beyond age eighty-five. "Life span," on the other hand, refers to the given amount of years a person lives, whether it is short or long. "Life span" in this sense is a neutral term, describing an overall duration of a person's life.

A study published in the medical journal *Lancet* in October 2009 found that if existing life expectancy trends continue, most babies born in the twenty-first century in Canada, France, Germany, Italy, Japan, the UK, the United States, and other developed countries with high life expectancy will live to at least one hundred years.[4]

In the same study, Professor Kaare Christensen and colleagues at the University of Southern Denmark write that half the babies born in the UK in 2007 will reach the age of 103, and half the babies born in Japan in the same year will live to be at least 107.[5]

A World Economic Forum report published in May 2017 predicted that the number of people worldwide aged sixty-five and older will exceed two billion by 2050.[6]

Because we will live longer, in the coming chapters we will discuss simple and practical tools that help us to stay in good health and remain disability free in our higher decades—in other words, how we can maintain our health span through our entire life span.

Remember what you represent, the limitless potential of existence. The energy and intelligence permeating the cosmos inform every cell in your body.

CHAPTER SEVEN

Evolution of the Mind

Following are three of countless examples throughout human history that illustrate the changing nature of what we believe to be possible at a certain period in time:

- Before Roger Bannister became the first human in 1954 to break the four-minute mile barrier, it was widely believed that no human would ever run a mile in under four minutes. It was considered physically impossible for humans to run at that speed. Bannister had run in the 1952 Helsinki Olympics and finished fourth in the 1,500 meters (slightly shorter than a mile). This below-par performance was a big disappointment for Bannister, and it drove him to develop his own training regimen of short, intense workout sessions to enable him to break the four-minute mark.

  On May 6, 1954, in Oxford, England, Bannister ran the mile in three minutes, 59.4 seconds. Following this groundbreaking feat, however, Bannister held the distinction of being the only human with below-four-minute-mile status for less than seven weeks. John Landy finished the mile in three minutes, 58 seconds on June 21, 1954, and another thirty-six people ran the mile in under four minutes by 1956. In the following nine years, more than 200 additional people did the same. What happened? A clear psychological barrier had been crossed. This was no longer considered impossible. Now it was brought inside the mental walls of what is considered doable.

The current world record in a mile, set in 1999 by Hicham El Guerrouj, stands at 3:43.13. What had been believed to be humanly impossible only forty-six years prior—which in the cosmic perspective is a blink of an eye—had now been reduced by seventeen seconds, which is a gigantic span in competitive running at this distance. A limit obviously exists, but where is it?

- After Orville and Wilbur Wright had begun flying their rudimentary airplanes at the beginning of the twentieth century, many people were afraid of going on a plane in person, but many also resisted the idea on philosophic principles: It was something that we humans were not meant to do. Their reasoning was that we are terrestrial creatures and as such should stay on the ground: birds belong in the sky, and humans belong on earth. Only one hundred years later, this type of thinking is clearly considered out-of-date.

- Readers over the age of fifty might marvel at the technological innovations of wearable computers, humanlike robots, and enhanced ebooks, but for people younger than twenty, this equipment is the only experience they've known. The processing power of computer chips is nearly doubling every eighteen months. The smartphone that fits in your hand has more computing power than the spacecraft *Apollo 11*, which landed on the moon in July 1969 for the first manned moonwalk of Neil Armstrong and Buzz Aldrin. That was the pinnacle of human ingenuity then; this you can now carry in your pocket. Today's children are born into this reality, and for them *this is normal.* So it is with any other novel information: At a certain point the extraordinary becomes routine, and then obsolete.

Ask yourself: What kind of limitations do I put on my own thinking? What do I presuppose from the start that I will not be able to do?

As described in Chapter 4, superstring theory shows the essence of the universe as made of packets of vibrating strings of potential, waves of probabilities, frequencies of information. We freeze a single outcome of an event into existence out of its various probabilities by the quality of our inner intention and the focus of our outward attention directed toward this object. This process begins in our minds, crystallizes into our thoughts, and manifests in reality through our actions.

And as was mentioned in Chapter 5, we live in a participatory universe. A different way of looking at it is that we are not only participants in our life, we are creators of our life. If we set out to do something we believe is impossible, we will have little likelihood of accomplishing this task. On the other hand, if we believe something is attainable by us, in that very realization lie the seeds of the successful outcome. The mathematical term for this is the *existence theorem*: Chances of finding a solution to a problem are greatly increased by the knowledge that a solution exists.

The deepest knowledge you can reach in this existence is self-awareness. When you understand yourself, you understand the world.

When we look at human history from a wide enough perspective we see that these transitions in perception of what is possible for us at a given time are a natural progression of knowledge. The world we live in today is clearly different from the world that existed 300, 3,000, and 3 million years ago. Change and evolution and further exploration are inherent features of existence. The ability to sense how long we can live is a latent capacity in us, currently unknown, as the introduction of fire, the invention of flying, and the discovery of radio waves were before we revealed them.

Shifts of Consciousness

Let's play a little mind game and travel back in time to England in the year 1545. Let's make you a successful and important person: You are a member of the court of King Henry VIII. You are well-respected and well-informed, and people seek your opinion on worldly matters.

One day a courier arrives at court with the news that a book written by scientist Nicolaus Copernicus says that Earth is not at the center of the world but somehow spins around the sun. *Ridiculous,* you think. *Who will believe this? Hang the heretic, or better yet torture him until he recants.* You at this time are not an ignorant person, you are just convinced that this idea is nonsense. Who can blame you?

Consider the shift in consciousness that this bizarre information required. The brightest minds on Earth had thought that all the planets and stars revolved around us. Day was day, and night was night. The stars were above in the heavens, and the sun rose in the east and set in the west, and the moon came on after darkness, and there was order in the world.

We have only traveled less than 500 years back. Let's jump back 500,000 years. What do we see? Rough life, harsh conditions. Now let's jump forward the same number of years. This entire expanse and more is your mental canvas, the evolutionary information contained in your genes.

It took 13.7 billion years for the universe to evolve from the moment of the big bang to the present moment of you reading this sentence. But the potential—the promise and the premise—of this moment existed right there at the moment of the big bang. Between the reality of the big bang and the reality of you reading this book are 13.7 billion years of chemical, physical, and biological processes; of planetary alignments; of temperature adjustments; and ongoing shifts of consciousness.

These two images in time—of the past "dark void" of the beginning of the universe and the present "ordered" world—are separated by billions of years of evolution. We have gone back 13.7 billion years. Let's now go forward that same distance. What can we see? It is safe to say that none of us can accurately predict that future world from our present station. This simple admission underscores the fact that the world we are observing today is not fixed and final, evolution keeps happening all the time; all matter—including you and me—is in constant flux.

The future is not the past. Time does not stop, nor does "life," the process of mutation, adaptation, transformation, and renewal. Existence consists of metabolism—that is, the breakdown of substance, absorption, conversion, assimilation, and fresh beginnings. This is the activity taking place in your body right at this moment, and right below the surface of every other object.

Because we are a product of the same cosmic forces that have created the universe we inhabit, we can see in ourselves the same universal laws that govern all existence in the cosmos. It's worth repeating that quantum mechanics derives its name from seeing the universe as composed of single indivisible units (*quanta,* the plural of *quantum*) of energy and matter, which adjust their behavior according to who is observing them and what their intention is. This innate flexibility and mutability are at the source of you and me, and the very essence of existence.

I personally have always needed to test any fancy idea I might have in the reality of daily life, and I will do the same here: Sitting in this chair writing this sentence, I am that chubby, innocent boy who got beat up at the age of ten walking home from school, but I'm not *just* that. Because the life I know best is my own, I'll use it here for illustration. I went through a phase of being a juvenile delinquent, and then a soldier, and then a private eye, and then a professional actor, and then I became an American citizen (and through all these phases remaining a loving son and brother), and now I am president of Lifespan Seminar and vice president of Asia Pacific Association of Psychology. I am the combination of all those things and more. I still have to live out my future. That will also end up being a part of my overall narrative. Why let a single past event define you? Why let your perception of yourself freeze at a certain point before you've completed your entire journey?

The universe doesn't stop evolving, and I don't stop from experiencing new things, so why should I freeze my identity at the age of ten, or thirty, or any other intermediary point along the journey? Life keeps happening and keeps affecting you.

By the same token, my genes contain the hereditary information of the single cell amoeba I had been along my evolutionary path, but not *just* that. Why fix your perception of yourself only at your past and present? They made you what you are, but that's not *all* you are. Why should you see that as the sum total of your existence?

These are understandable labels and identities that we assume in the natural cycle of life. The traditional way of looking at this passage from one phase to another is reinventing yourself, but a more accurate view is coming to know yourself. By going through these different incarnations you discover your true self. Through all these experiences you peel the outer layers of your existence to arrive at your core. What resonates with you the most? What can't you help doing? How do you define yourself? When you address yourself, who is the *I* that answers?

What is your essence? My essence is being an explorer, of myself and life. Stretching the boundaries of what it means to be alive and to be human. My primary obligation is to live out the 102-year duration that has been shown to me, and to put that time to the best use. What is the use? Grasp the enormity and limitless possibilities of existence and of our own individual infinite powers, and communicate these to others in a way that they can use to improve their own lives.

Here's the true mental challenge: Can you have a view of yourself that incorporates your entire span of existence? Can you step back and have a vision of your life that includes what you have been in the past, what you are today, and also all the promise of your future? Can you see the vast potential inherent in your genes and make it come true?

Don't be afraid to be what you are capable of being.

Our Future Selves

As we saw at the beginning of this chapter with the example of Roger Bannister breaking the four-minute barrier in the mile, throughout human history breakthroughs regularly occur in which a previous threshold has been transcended, and following which a new concept of reality has been formed. A similar phenomenon is evident every time an especially gifted athlete emerges on the scene. Michael Jordan transformed existing notions of human capacity beyond the game of basketball. Watching him hover in the air on his way to a dunk was an inspiring experience. Seeing another human perform a remarkable feat helps us locate that same potential in ourselves. Clearly not at the same level of competence and execution, but an experience of this nature opens a mental window in our psyche to dormant attributes we didn't know existed. What had been previously thought impossible is now accepted as possible, as a new benchmark by which to measure other activities is assimilated into our collective consciousness. Usain Bolt's running at the Beijing and London Olympics electrified the audience and again brought into question where the limits of human abilities might be.

From an evolutionary perspective, this is what we humans have always done and will continue doing: exploring our minds and bodies for the latent powers inherent in our genes.

Latent dictionary definition:

1. Present and capable of becoming though not now visible or active.
2. Power or quality that has not yet come forth but may emerge and develop.
3. (Psychoanalysis) present but unexpressed: present in the unconscious but not consciously expressed.
4. (Biology) dormant: undeveloped but able to develop normally under suitable conditions.

For you to be able to locate in your mind and body the awareness of your optimal duration will require a shift in consciousness. You, as an individual, are the result of everything you've done up to this point; everything you've thought; and every action you took and refrained from taking. On the collective level, you are the descendant of the hominid who first figured how to tame fire; domesticate the horse and the dog; and you are at the present stage of evolution because of the contributions of Copernicus, Galileo, Newton, and also Steve Jobs and Elon Musk.

You are a culmination of everything that came before you, and in you there is a promise of everything that will come.

Each thing that any of us can do, every one of us is capable of doing *in potentia*. We are individual manifestations of the cosmic whole—the consciousness permeating the universe. Our personalities consist of the same ingredients in different proportions. Some of us have more courage, or more mathematical skills, or better physical ability as part of our inherited makeup, but we all have all those components in varying degrees. By focusing our attention on a particular capacity, we can enhance it and multiply it. When a new ability is added to the shared vocabulary of human existence, that potential becomes available to every member of the species.

Just one hundred years ago, the most advanced science of the time thought that the universe consisted of a single galaxy, the Milky Way, in the midst of a vast, dark, infinite, empty space. This is what we could see with the most sophisticated telescopes of the day. A century later, our latest telescopes help us understand that we are living in an expanding universe of which we can only see 5 percent, whereas the nature of the remaining 95 percent is yet beyond our knowledge.

This fact illustrates once again that evolution never stops; it's taking place here and now, where I am and where you are. Existence equals evolution. As long as we and the universe exist we will be going through our biological processes of growth and decline, metabolism, discovery and learning; and the universe will be going through its cosmological processes of stars forming and dying, planetary alignments, and temperature adjustments. Of course, the big bang itself, and what will happen at the end of the world, is also a part of this evolutionary process. Evolution, in its purest sense, means moving from one stage to another.

In his 2013 book *A Universe from Nothing*, Lawrence Krauss, professor at the School of Earth and Space Exploration at the department of physics at Arizona State University, details the latest discoveries of cosmology and physics to describe the universe emerging from "nothingness" before the big bang, to a possible time two trillion years forward when astronomers of the far future will have no clue of the past existence of the four hundred billion galaxies in our currently visible universe, because the evidence will have disappeared. Our expanding universe will have stretched so far that those distant galaxies are no longer visible.[1]

That is the impermanent universe we presently occupy. However, the focus of this book is not cosmology but helping you to live your longest and healthiest life. We accept the outer impermanence surrounding our existence and present the stable center on which we can rely in our individual lives. Where is that center? In me. In you. In knowing what makes your body feel good and healthy. In knowing what gives you meaning, satisfaction, and pleasure. In knowing love, affection, and fulfillment. In the midst of all that uncertainty, we are not lost. We are not helpless. We accept the transitory character of our existence, and we take responsibility for our own well-being. This is not insignificant. This is the making of a full, good life.

Another open question that neuroscience, philosophy, medicine, and other branches of science presently face is a definition of the mind that can be acceptable across the different disciplines. Just like a clear and inclusive definition of consciousness, that is still a work in progress. Although most researchers agree that the likeliest place in the body to look for the mind is the brain, recent studies show that that could not be the *only* area where the mind is located. Your mind is in all the cells of your body. The entire body serves as the mind, as an entity that senses, feels, gathers, and transmits information.

One workable definition of the mind that has been emerging is instead of thinking of it as an object and pinning it down in a particular area of the body, it's better thought of as a process that controls the flow of energy and information through the body.

Latest neuroscience research shows that we have complex, adaptive, and functional neural networks, or "brains," in our heart and gut. The "heart brain" is called the cardiac nervous system, and the "gut brain" is called enteric nervous system. These adaptive neural systems exhibit extraordinary capacities for memory and intuitive intelligence. In addition, there's increasing evidence that these brains located in our heart and gut play a key role in processing physical and mental functions.

Because we've already seen in Chapter 5 that the mind—this mental process—controls the body, we can assimilate this new awareness that the mind regulates the distribution of energy throughout the body. This means understanding the amount and quality of the energy contained in your body, and then making conscious choices on how to use this energy on the life path you've chosen for yourself.

CHAPTER EIGHT

Wisdom of the Body

In your body, the entire universe is contained. The knowledge is not "out there," it is in here.

In the preceding chapters we saw the most recent discoveries that modern science gives us on how our mind works. Let's now look at the human body to see exactly how *it* works. Our body is a well-designed machine for living with built-in mechanisms for self-healing and self-correction, provided we don't harm it with bad habits.

The human body is also the most sophisticated pharmacological lab in existence. The body contains forty trillion cells working in remarkable agreement to keep it in the best condition.[1] Through long evolution, it perfected its ability to fight off diseases and balance its internal processes. It does this through a natural state called "homeostasis," or self-regulation, during which it maintains biological processes, hormonal stability, and internal temperature within an optimal range. The body intuitively knows how to take care of itself. For example, we sweat to cool off during hot summer days, and we shiver to produce heat during cold winter months.

So the answer to the natural question of "How do you know how long you could live?" is this: The body knows. Just like we know when we're hungry, tired, or cold, when we develop a higher awareness of our physical and mental states, we gain access to our body's intuition, which is the age-old wisdom inherent in our genes.

The human body is a celestial body, informed with cosmic consciousness. When you access your body's intuition you access universal intelligence.

The latest research of Rudolph Tanzi, professor of neurology at Harvard University, indicates that intuition is the next big part of the brain that is evolving, as it relates to the mind: the instinctive brain followed by the emotional brain, followed by the intellectual brain, and next the intuitive brain.[2] In this understanding, intuition is not merely a reflexive behavior we've been conditioned for, as the early instinctive stage of our brain was. Intuition is a culmination of all our qualities of intelligence, vision, self-knowledge, and knowledge of the world—mind, body, and soul.

In Chapter 7 we saw that our mind is responsible for regulating our body, but it is also a part of our body. Our entire body feels, senses, thinks, collects, and transmits information. There is an ongoing feedback loop between the body and the brain. This is a key feature of the mind-body interaction: The body sends signals to the brain about its current needs and condition. The region in our brain above the sockets of the eyes is called the orbitofrontal cortex. This brain region's primary function is integrating the continuous signals coming in from the body about the state that the body is in, whether it's excited, hungry, thirsty, embarrassed, or happy.[3]

Your emotional states affect your physical condition, and vice versa. Rather than see a division between mind and body, this a good place to start looking at this process as the unity of mind-body-energy operation. This is the entirety of your conscious organism. As Norman Doidge writes in *The Brain that Changes Itself*:

> We have long viewed our imaginative life with a kind of sacred awe: as noble, pure, immaterial, and ethereal, cut off from our material brain. Now we cannot be so sure about where to draw the line between them. Everything your "immaterial" mind imagines leaves material traces. Each thought alters the physical state of your brain synapses at a microscopic level. Each time you

imagine moving your fingers across the keys to play the piano, you alter the tendrils in your living brain.[4]

Most of the mental activity in the body takes place in the brain, which is the control center of your whole system. The mind is connected to the brain, and the brain is part of the body. Although during our daily lives we are not aware of this occurrence, our physical body changes all the time. In a year we recycle 98 percent of matter in the body and in less than two years our body totally rebuilds itself. Every cell in our body eventually dies and is replaced by new cells. Our body builds a whole new skeleton in three months. Our brain rebuilds itself in one year. Our liver re-creates itself in six weeks. Our skin rebuilds itself in one year. Our blood renews itself in four months. Our stomach lining rebuilds itself in five days. And our entire DNA renews itself every two months.

An important awareness to take from these facts is to live in this particular body we currently have: understand it, come to terms with it, and take responsibility for it. Not trying to be what we were 10 years ago or last year—because that is not possible—but creating the best conditions for this body here and now. Some people live primarily in their minds and neglect to acknowledge their bodies. Since we are made of flesh, blood, and bones, life is not only a mental experience but, first and foremost, a physical one.

Exercise: Body Awareness

Note: As mentioned before, I recommend that you first read each exercise aloud as you record your voice, and then play it back. This way, you don't need to hold the book to follow the instructions.

Lie or sit down in your favorite place, and make yourself comfortable and relaxed.

Drop in and concentrate on your breath. Make sure it is steady and free. Inhale, exhale—nice and easy, deep, effortless, even breaths. Breath is the key to your body. It is the door by which you enter your inner world. Take the time to establish a stable pattern of breaths.

Do not rush with the following sequence or anticipate any outcome. Simply visit each part of your body as you begin a mental checklist, and pay close attention to the condition of each part you visit. Begin with the limbs that are farthest away from your head:

How do my toes feel?

How do my ankles feel?

My calves? Shins? Knees? Thighs?

Continue moving upward in your body to reach your head.

Move your jaw and notice if it feels tight or loose.

If it feels tight, breathe into this area, and energize it by lightly massaging it as you mentally release the tension that is stored in that spot.

Continue with other parts:

How do my ears feel? My forehead? My nose?

Gently massage your scalp with your hands.

Move down and massage your face, chin, and cheeks.

As you do this, listen to and sense the underlying rhythm of your body. This is your internal engine: your heartbeat, your breath, your lungs expanding and contracting.

What you're doing with these activities is getting familiar with your primary home—your body—in the most direct manner. Once you've established a steady, even breath pattern and your body feels relaxed, begin to meditate on the following topics:

I am as much a drop in the cosmic ocean of existence as this entire ocean is contained in me. My DNA contains the energy and information of the cosmos, everything that's happened, is happening, and will happen.

Energy is that which has the capacity to move things.

Information is data and facts.

By trusting my body's intuition, I trust universal intelligence.

My body is a self-contained structure in time and space.

My heartbeat is an offshoot of the pulse of the universe. And my bloodstream carries the life force which drives all things in the cosmos.

The body I inhabit—skin, flesh, and bones—is an independent sphere within a larger environment. The same cosmic forces that influence events in the universe also govern my body.

I am an hourglass of potential, a vessel into which various characteristics, skills, capacities, and attributes have been poured.

I am also an hourglass in time and space, a product of everything that happened in the universe before I was born.

A portion of time inhabits and passes through my body: the past entering when I am born, staying in present reality as long as I live, and moving into the future when I pass on.

I come from the source of life, and I return to the source of life when I complete my life cycle.

Going through the cycle of life and growing older is not a detriment but a natural process like seasonal weather, and I can approach it with the same attitude. Since I cannot prevent one or the other, what I can do is adapt and learn how to be the best version of myself at every age with the choices I make in everyday life.

Stay in this realization as you breathe steady and free, and make sure your body is relaxed and comfortable.

Use this mantra to see how your daily actions fit in the larger framework: One choice at a time, one action at a time, and before you know it, it ends up being your life.

Now slowly bring this exercise to an end. Get up from the floor with the least amount of effort and rejoin your day.

In previous chapters, we also described the essential makeup of the universe and saw that the human body is made of the same ingredients as everything else in the cosmos. We saw that the consciousness that permeates the universe is the same life force that drives our bodies. We went billions of years back to the presently understood origins of the world at the big bang, and we gazed far into the future to envision the entire span of evolution.

Going forward, we will bring this sense of the world at large back into our inner world by beginning to recognize the processes taking place in our bodies. This means coming to recognize and trust our body's intuition, and relying on the signals that the body is sending us continuously about what makes for a healthy and optimal life.

We will begin to learn how to create in our daily life the conditions where we feel at our best physically, mentally, and emotionally. We will also see how to gauge the quality and the quantity of the energy coursing through your body and how to use it in the manner that you choose.

Your body is never static, never set in stone.

Like the universe itself, it experiences mutation, evolution, progress.

The wisdom in your body is the wisdom of the world.

PART THREE

Mastering the Mind
and Body

Body consciousness = cosmic consciousness.
In your body, the entire universe is contained. Your body knows.

CHAPTER NINE

Body Consciousness Techniques

Mindfulness

For the sake of clarity and simplicity, let's first define the term *mindfulness*. Mindfulness basically means living with attention, not doing things thoughtlessly or on autopilot. It's being aware, being present in the moment, being in charge of your actions, knowing why you do what you, rather than sleep-walking through life.

Although in the last few years mindfulness has become a hot topic, being practiced in universities, corporations, prisons, sport teams, and high schools, many people still think of it as a rather obscure Eastern practice that has something to do with sitting cross-legged and chanting.

Rather than having scheduled sessions of mindfulness at given times, true mindfulness is something that you experience all the time: You go through your life in a state of mindfulness. This wakes you up to existence, gives you responsibility and authority over your life, and helps you make conscientious choices. You are living an awakened life, walking the path that you've laid for yourself.

Mindfulness also means the state of being in harmony among your mind, body, and the universe. It is a way to come to know yourself, and when your mind understands itself it understands the world. This mind has come to know what it can control and what is beyond its control. A mind at peace accepts all the things it can't control, because fighting them is a waste of energy, and energy, like time, is a precious and finite commodity.

With the hectic modern lifestyles that most of us experience, there's an onslaught of good and bad information assaulting our senses all the time. Since the dawn of the digital age, the human attention span has shrunk from twelve seconds to only eight seconds.[1] Meditation is a technique that helps you achieve mindfulness. The way to access your center is by quieting the background noise. In meditation, when you quell the noise in the brain you open the channels of intuition, your innate mechanism of knowing right from wrong, foresight, and wisdom.

Meditation

Buddha was asked, "What have you gained from meditation?" "Nothing," he replied. "However, I'll tell you what I've lost: anger, anxiety, depression, insecurity, fear of old age, and death."

We begin body consciousness techniques with meditation because this is a practice that most people have heard about even if they've never done it. Eastern spiritual traditions have known about the benefits of meditation for millennia. In the past few decades, Western-led science has added to this understanding with studies that document the clear effects that meditation has on our overall health. Here is the shortest way to describe how meditation improves our well-being: Meditation calms the mind, which calms the body, which enables the body to regain its balance.

Although essentially body and mind are inseparable for establishing a healthy lifestyle, in this part of the book we will focus on developing consciousness that is primarily located in the body, and in the following parts we will cover practical skills and mental imagery tools that are mainly triggered in the mind.

It's worth pointing out that the words *medicine* and *meditation* are linked at the root. They come from Latin: "to cure." The word also carries the meaning of measuring, as in taking stock of our inner state, understanding our mind and body.

It is useful to consider the two key dictionary definitions of meditation because they help us access in ourselves the portals by which we pass into a deeper understanding of our inner world:

Empty or concentrate mind: to empty the mind of thoughts, or concentrate the mind on one thing, in order to aid mental or spiritual development, contemplation, or relaxation.

Think carefully about something: to think about something carefully, calmly, seriously, and for some time.

The more in-depth ways in which mindfulness and meditation affect your well-being include:

- Increase activity in different brain regions, including those responsible for emotion regulation, learning, and memory, and seeing things from a wider perspective.
- Relieve psychological conditions such as anxiety, phobias, insomnia, and eating disorders.
- Improve psychological functions of concentration, compassion, attention, and empathy.
- Boost the immune system.
- Improve medical conditions, such as cardiovascular disease, asthma, premenstrual syndrome, type 2 diabetes, and chronic pain.

General Guidelines to Help You Get the Most out of Meditation Exercises

Choose a place where you will not be disturbed and where you can control the environment: the amount of light, the level of noise, your favorite temperature, and so forth. The goal is to create conditions in which you can be as relaxed and focused as possible. As you become more proficient with these exercises, you will be able to do them as you go about your daily life in every environment, even in loud and crowded places. However, at the beginning it is important to establish the most favorable circumstances for your quick mastery of these techniques.

Allow yourself twenty- to forty-minute installments as you begin doing these exercises. Our aim here is to demystify these meditation sessions. Other people do them, and you can do them as well—with fun and pleasure. You want to dedicate at least twenty minutes to each session in order for your mind-body connection to develop responsiveness and awareness. If you can fit a forty-minute session in your daily routine, it is recommended for significant progress. But don't worry if that's not possible. A twenty-minute session once a day will result in significant benefits.

Remember: Not every exercise is right for you, nor will you resonate with each exercise. Your increasing self-mastery will come from starting to identify what works for you, and then incorporating those exercises into an easy routine in your daily life, in a way that fits comfortably with your energy and schedule.

Don't be too harsh on yourself if you don't detect a noticeable change in your body and mind right away. In this context it is good to use the analogy of the tango: two steps forward and one step back, which is the natural learning curve for every new skill. Keep telling yourself this is a lifelong habit that will benefit you—for life. At a certain point you will start wondering how you could previously do without these enjoyable routines.

As you become more and more familiar with each individual exercise, it's quite likely that you'll develop your personal set of exercises out of the ones described in this book, which will combine effortlessly with your individual rhythm and lifestyle. Trust this process and trust your body. Your body holds vast reservoirs of wisdom and will reveal them to you as you become more confident and attentive to its needs.

The biggest reason why people give up their New Year's resolutions is that they feel a sense of burden, a restriction imposed on their lives. For you to assimilate new healthy habits in your life permanently, your most important transformation is to do them not as a chore but a choice. You'll do these exercises not because someone told you to, but because they'll make you feel good, and enable you to be at your optimal condition at every age, which is a gift you give to yourself.

At the center of chaos and uncertainty there's peace. This peace resides inside you.

Exercise: Meditation on Abundance

Lie or sit down in your favorite place, make yourself comfortable, and establish a free, deep, and steady pattern of breaths.

Run a quick mental checklist through your limbs to assess the overall feeling of your body.

See if you want to adjust your body, stretch, yawn, or roll your shoulders to loosen up.

When you feel a free flow of energy in your body, begin directing your attention to each separate limb. Start farthest away from your head.

Wiggle the toes of your left foot several times to establish freedom and ease.

Do the same with the toes of your right foot.

Now move your focus up to your ankles. Picture in your mind your left ankle as a supple joint moving easily without obstruction.

Repeat this process with your right ankle.

Once you've determined that both your ankles are pliant, move your attention up to your calves (first left, then right), then to your shins and knees, as you repeat the same procedure at every station and take your time, not rushing any stage.

Move in this way through each part of your body rising higher toward your pelvis, abdomen, chest, and shoulders.

Now go down to your arms, elbows, and hands.

Move the fingers of your left hand gently to see that they are not holding any tension. Do the same with your right hand. Shake both your hands lightly and exhale simultaneously to release any remaining residue of tightness.

Now slowly move back toward your head. Draw into your center and ask yourself:

- Am I comfortable in this position?
- Do I need to move slightly to the left or right to feel better in my body?
- Is there anything I can improve right now to feel looser? Freer? More at ease?

If the answer is yes, do just that.

Now go down to your chin, then your neck, and enter your chest cavity to access your heart.

Make sure your breath is steady, easy, and plentiful.

Grow quiet at the center of your heart as you breathe deeply, evenly, and calmly.

Now imagine a glowing sun sitting at the center of your heart. It fills you with a warm radiance of light and pleasure. Sense it spreading in all directions through your chest, ribs, and back, soaking each area with bright and vital energy as it moves through every limb. As the morning sun glows increasingly more intense when it rises in the sky, this heat is reaching further through your body—all the way to your fingers, calves, toes, and shoulders, and the top of your head.

Now there is fluid and potent energy flowing through every part of your body. Stay in this glow for several minutes, enjoying the state of relaxation and suppleness washing through your whole body.

Meditate on this feeling of abundance and at the same time acknowledge the blessings in your life. Count them in your mind. What are you grateful for:

A loving relationship?

Your health and the health of your loved ones?

Your job?

Your home?

Notice every significant item in your life that makes you feel happy and safe.

Relax and register this feeling of gratitude washing through every area in your body.

You want to retain this sensation of light, peace, and richness as you slowly begin to wrap this exercise and rejoin your daily routine.

As you revisit this exercise on a regular basis, this sense of affluence, security, and well-being will gradually become the default condition of your life.

These meditation routines help you develop a new perception of your entire being. Your body becomes more responsive, more resonant, and more alive. You discover new understandings and new wisdom in your body. A new license and responsibility reveal themselves to you—to solely do what agrees with your health, and not do anything that harms your well-being. You reveal a sense of order, correlation, and agreement among the different parts of your body. You begin to see that *you are this body*; the person that you are and the life that you have are a clear reflection of your physical being.

Meditation also lets you access your higher self: your best traits, capacities, and intentions. It awakens your better angels. Buddha expressed a similar thought 2,600 years ago when he said, "Meditation is a way for nourishing and blossoming the divinity within you."

As you gradually become more familiar with meditation you can use it to improve your approach to every aspect of your existence: work, health, family, finances, and romance. These deep relaxation sessions are the ideal setting for your imagination, intuition, and problem-solving skills to emerge and apply in your everyday life.

A useful mantra: *Slow down, don't rush. Find something to enjoy in this moment.*

Pressure Points

Pressure points are powerful and convenient tools to gain awareness and control of your body, as well as helping the body release tension and realign itself. The pressure points are considered direct doorways to accessing your body's neural networks. There are more than seventy pressure points throughout the human body. The most easily accessible ones are on your forehead, under your earlobes, in your eye sockets, on the palms, and in the webs between your fingers.

Our nervous system consists of a neural grid that connects the different parts of the body. When there is a knot or an energy block somewhere in this network it registers as little lumps in the pressure points on your face, on your head, and on the palms of your hands. You can relieve them by massaging these pressure points that are easily accessible with your fingers, and this will release those blockages to resume a free flow of energy through your body.

These natural energy points are located along meridians, or pathways that crisscross the head, arms, legs, and trunk. These meridians are channels through which the body's energy (what Chinese medicine calls Qi, or life force, or vital energy) flows through the body. When this vital energy flow is low or restricted, the body becomes unbalanced, which suppresses its immune system.

As an illustration of their centrality in the body, because these pressure points are direct portals into the nervous system, martial artists who have studied the locations of the pressure points through the body can quickly disable attackers by using a simple but focused push on a pressure point on the head, the neck, or in the trunk.

Your body is a repository of everything you experience: elation, sadness, frustration, fear, pain, love, hate, exhaustion, jubilation, and stress. Stress can be defined as anything that knocks your body out of its natural rhythm. Everything that happens in the mind has a correlate in the body. This regular storing of mental information in the body is done both consciously and subconsciously. The psyche protects itself by suppressing deeply unpleasant episodes in the subconscious, and these unwelcome incidents may resurface when a present analogous event triggers the buried past memory. The body may retain stress and pain to such an extent that sometimes an entire area of the body can be blocked and result in restricted mobility.

There are two main types of blockages in the body: mental and physical. The former may be caused by repressed negative occasions, and the latter by past bodily injuries and ailments. Either type can cause blockages in energy flow. Pressure points help you to release the tension that your body regularly accumulates through the day, and this leads to a free flow of energy in the body and enables the body to restore its equilibrium.

Exercise: Pressure Points

Using your thumb, forefinger, and middle finger gently begin applying pressure in your lower forehead just above the eyebrows. Lightly massage the middle of your forehead, while you direct your breaths to the place where your fingers touch the skin. This may result in deep sighs, which is a sign that your body is releasing stress and readjusting itself. Once you feel comfortable with this activity, close your eyes and continue doing it for thirty seconds. Keep your breaths steady, even, and free, and pay attention to the reactions generated in your body. This may prompt you to stretch your shoulders, rotate your neck, or exhale and inhale deeply. These are all natural signals that your body is realigning itself. Do this for as long as it's comfortable.

Next, using only the tip of your forefinger, lightly poke under your earlobe in the dip where it meets the jaw and the neck. This little crater is one of the most sensitive spots in the body. It is a direct access to the body's neural system. You can close your eyes and do this for another minute or longer if you like, as you let go of any tension that might be in your body. Focus on your breath to make sure that it is steady and free, and see if you want to readjust yourself by gently moving your shoulders, neck, or jaw.

Now, using only your thumb and forefinger, start applying pressure in the upper inner corners of your eye sockets, on either side of your nose bridge, right below the eyebrows, where the nose meets your forehead. Gently rub this area in a circular motion. There are little dips there on either side of your nose bridge, and these are the points where you want to apply light pressure with the tips of your thumb and your forefinger. As you do this, direct your breaths to where your fingers touch your skin, and again make sure that your breaths are free, steady, and deep. Close your eyes and do this for another minute or longer if you like. It might be that the release of tension in your body that this activity generates will prompt you to continue doing this for several minutes. The benefits of pressure points can be both immediate and significant.

Next, using your thumb and forefinger, gently pinch the web between your pinky and ring finger on your other hand. Do this for a while, and then go a little further up and explore the space between the knuckles of your hand by gently massaging there and feeling for possible lumps. When you locate one of these lumps, start applying light pressure to it with your thumb and forefinger. This might also prompt deep sighs or exhalations, which are a sign of your body releasing pent-up energy and stress. The body regularly stores tension in these spots, and what you're doing now is releasing those energy knots.

Now use the same thumb and forefinger to investigate the other webs between your fingers to see if there are any lumps. Sometimes it can feel like a dim pain or local sensitivity in the area. When you discover a lump, start gently kneading it with your thumb and forefinger to disperse that pent-up energy in the body. You can apply as much pressure as you like, and go as deep as you like, without causing pain or discomfort.

Next, go up to the center of your palm and gently explore the whole surface of your palm and back of hand to see if there are any energy knots there. You can also use your thumb, forefinger, and middle finger, if that's more comfortable for you, as shown in the picture on the next page. Next, go down to the sides of your fingers and gently pinch the skin with your thumb and forefinger to see if you feel any knots. Knead that entire area with your fingers and remember to breathe deep breaths.

Switch hands and do the same on the other hand. Some of these lumps can be really hard. If there's significant stress stored in that spot that place can feel raw or tender, and it might hurt a bit when you massage the area. You want to apply just the right amount of pressure to relieve this knot without causing any harm. Moderate pain that you can tolerate is a positive sign of the tension in the spot slowly starting to melt as you knead this lump in a circular motion.

Switch between your hands and continue doing this for another few minutes. Make sure that you're breathing steady and free, and notice the reactions generated in your body. These energy lumps are now slowly being released and dissolved into your blood stream like salt in water.

Now, we'll slowly bring this exercise to an end. Feels good, right? You've just released some pent-up stress that was accumulated in your body.

As these handy routines show, you can do these pressure points without calling unnecessary attention to yourself as you go about your everyday life. The five pressure point locations on your body described here are easily accessible in most circumstances in our daily routines. You can do them while walking, driving, at your desk, sitting in the bus, on your lunch break, and in front of a TV. They are perfect for relieving headaches, to stabilize your heartbeat, to help restore better blood flow through the body, and to help you deal with anxieties and stressful situations.

Ring Muscles

The human body contains a system of muscles that regulate the basic functions of existence. These are called the ring muscles because they are round and are located around every opening in the body, both internally and externally. The ring muscles' natural pattern of simultaneous contraction and relaxation is responsible for a harmonious operation of the entire body.

The ring muscles, also called sphincters, are at the core of every form of animal life, from the plainest amoeba to the most complex human body. They are among the earliest systems in any living organism, and they are joined to the primal part of the human brain, the spinal cord, which is the neural chassis of the body. The ring muscles control reproduction and self-preservation, heart regulation, blood circulation, digestion and elimination, respiration, and all other muscular coordination through the body.

When we are born all these muscles work together, releasing and contracting at the same time. That's the normal condition of the body. That's why a baby's fists are clenched. As we grow older, we develop bad habits. We slouch as we walk, we stick our guts out, we sit in bad postures, and all these behaviors short-circuit the network of communication signals between and among the different systems of the body and cause the body to fall out of alignment. This in turn harms the digestive processes, the blood flow, and the immune system. Ring muscles boost the body's immune system because the contractions and releases routines stimulate a better blood flow and an adequate supply of oxygen in the body.

Though there are more than fifty different sphincters in the human body (including around eyes, ears, nostrils, the mouth, the urethra, and the anus), the most important ones to the body's optimal operation are the lower sphincters: front sphincter (of the urethra) and rear sphincter (of the anus). The lower sphincters are vital to the proper functioning of the body because they are located at the gravitational center of the body—the midsection—and their contraction and relaxation cycles support every movement that we make. Our mouth opens and closes to eat and drink. Our hands open and close to hold and let go. Our heart contracts and relaxes to pump blood through the body. The stomach and intestines contract and relax to metabolize food.

This pattern of contraction and release in our bodies is an aspect of the elemental principle of duality underlying all life in the universe: darkness and light, death and birth, male and female, yin and yang. This is another way in which the natural laws of the universe govern the human body.

In a healthy body, all the sphincters work together, contracting and relaxing at the same time. The ring muscles are ultimately responsible for putting all the other muscles and all the organs of the body to work in a harmonious manner. It is good to remember that the human body is a well-designed system programmed for self-healing and self-correction, provided we don't harm it with bad habits and allow its natural processes to operate without obstruction.

Some sphincters are visible to the naked eye and some can only be seen with a microscope. As noted, they regulate the body's integrated operation throughout and also essential local functions:

- The microscopic precapillary sphincters control the blood flow into capillaries as part of the body's metabolic activity.
- The lower esophageal sphincter (the cardiac sphincter in the upper stomach) prevents the acidic contents of the stomach from moving upward into the esophagus.
- The sphincter of Oddi allows secretions to pass from the gallbladder, liver, and pancreas into the duodenum, the first segment of the small intestine.
- The ileocecal sphincter (at the junction of the small intestine and the large intestine) limits the reflux of colonic contents back into the ileum, the lowest section of the small intestine.

Some ring muscles are voluntary, meaning we can activate them at will, and some are involuntary, part of the body's autonomic nervous system, over which we have no control. We begin the ring muscles exercise with the sphincter where you have the most initial control, in your mouth.

Exercise: Ring Muscles

The exercises listed here restore the innate balance of the body by gradually re-establishing the original coordination of the different ring muscles. By deliberately initiating contractions and releases of the sphincters, you prompt the ring muscles to recover their unified activity through the body, which resets the entire body to its original equilibrium.

At the beginning, allow twenty minutes for this session. As your body develops awareness of this process, and you start to notice improvements in your body alignment, your digestive cycle, and a better energy flow in your body, you will want to increase the duration of the exercises to thirty minutes at a time, for the simple reason that they make you feel good, balanced, and rejuvenated.

Every time you do these exercises there is work done both on your body and your mind. Your conscious decision to attend to your body's well-being clearly translates to your mental realm; you derive a clear benefit from knowing that you're doing everything in your power to create the conditions where you can be at your very best. *This is all you can do—and it's plenty.*

As you begin these exercises keep in mind that eventually all your ring muscles will operate in their original unison. We start the process of restoring this fundamental harmony in your body by accessing the system through the easiest opening, and where you have the most control: through your mouth.

First Session

Lie down on your back and bring forward your legs to your chest, as you support yourself by holding your palms on your knees, or on your shins, in order to maintain this position comfortably with the least amount of effort.

Make sure you're not holding any tension in your neck, jaw, or shoulders.

If you feel tension somewhere, breathe deeply into that place and let go of the stress.

Roll from side to side to iron your lower back against the floor, which releases pressure between the vertebrae in the bottom of your spinal cord and ensures that the spinal cord stays flexible and healthy for years to come.

Bring yourself to a spot where you can comfortably stay in this position for as long as you like.

Once you're comfortable, begin gently contracting your mouth: Contract (pucker up), hold, release. Contract, hold, release.

Do this five times and rest.

Now do it ten more times and rest.

Simply contract, hold, release; contract, hold, release.

Don't expect or anticipate any major developments at this time. Allow your body the time it needs to restore itself to its original balance.

Rest, and do another set of ten.

Release your legs to the floor and rest in this comfortable position for several minutes. This is an important part of the exercise because now you are allowing this new awareness to assimilate throughout your body.

What you've started by triggering the ring muscles in your mouth is now registering in the different parts of your body.

You might notice deep sighs, an urge to stretch your arms, or wiggle your toes, or a feeling of shifting alignments through your body, all of which mean that your body is releasing accumulated tension. Don't force anything. Simply absorb this new feeling in your body.

Once this phase has run its course, bring your legs back up, supporting them with your palms on the knees or shins.

Begin by contracting your mouth and now also add your eyes—with the same motion, puckering (contracting) your mouth and squeezing (contracting) your eyes at the same time.

Contract, hold, release.

Repeat this with both mouth and eyes five times.

Rest.

Do the same set five times.

Rest.

Do the same set ten times. Make sure to maintain steady and free breaths.

Release your legs to the floor and rest.

This will conclude your first session. Roll from left to right and back to feel a free flow of energy in your body, and then slowly rise from the floor with the least possible effort.

When you are completely up, stand quietly and draw into your center. Notice how the different parts of your body feel: your legs, groin area, abdomen, chest, back, and head. Now slowly move forward and rejoin your daily routine.

To get the most benefit from this exercise it's best to do it at least twice a week. This way your body is able to build on the progress of the last session, without too many days lapsing in between.

If you can do thirty-minute sessions, your body will really appreciate it. But even fifteen to twenty minutes a couple times a week will do you a lot of good.

Second Session

Lie down on your back and bring forward your legs, helping to support yourself by holding your palms on your knees or shins, in order to comfortably maintain this position for as long as you like.

Begin by gently contracting your mouth and eyes at the same time: Contract, hold, release. Contract, hold, release.

Repeat this process five times, keeping even breaths as you go.

Rest.

Do the same set ten times.

Rest.

Repeat ten times.

Bring your legs down to the floor and rest.

Once this relaxation and assimilation phase has run its course, bring your legs back up, supporting them with your palms on the knees or shins.

Now begin by contracting you mouth, eyes, and also add your nostrils, all at the same time: puckering (contracting) your mouth, and squeezing (contracting) your eyes and nostrils simultaneously.

Contract, hold, release.

Repeat five times.

Rest.

Do another set of five.

Rest.

Do the same set ten times. Make sure to maintain steady and free breaths.

As you continue to do these sequences, you'll notice that your ears also join in the action. You have less control in your ears than in the first three sphincters you've been using, but as your body regains its original unison, your ears simply get pulled into the cycle.

Repeat another set of set contractions and releases.

Release your legs to the floor and rest.

You will conclude this session the same way as the last: rising from the floor with the least amount of effort. When you're standing on your feet, draw into your center, and roll your head gently, first to one side then the other. Now you're ready to rejoin your day.

Do the combinations of mouth, eyes, nostrils, and ears several times. When you feel ready to move forward, you will add to these sets your front and back sphincters.

Third Session: Lower Sphincters

To understand the mechanism at work in this exercise, there is an external urethral sphincter over which we have control, and an internal urethral sphincter, over which we have no control. When we initiate the constriction and release of the external sphincter, that pulls into the unified contraction-and-release routine the internal sphincter as well.

The urethral sphincter controls the urinary bladder to the urethra, the tube that drains urine from the body. Like the urethral sphincter, there is an external and internal anal sphincter, the former under our voluntary control, and the latter, part of the body's autonomic nervous system, outside of our direct control, but that gets pulled into the overall muscle contraction activity by the other muscles we initiate.

Lie down on your back and bring your knees up toward your chest, helping to support yourself by holding your palms on your knees or shins, in order to maintain this position comfortably for as long as you like.

Begin by gently contracting your mouth, eyes, nostrils, and ears simultaneously: Contract, hold, release. Contract, hold, release.

Repeat five times, keeping even breaths as you go.

Rest.

Now add your front sphincter, contracting it at the same time as you contract your other sphincters. The sense is of all five working effortlessly together.

The first times you use the front sphincter in this exercise it might feel like when you hold yourself from going to the bathroom. This is normal and a sign that your sphincter is now participating in the original unison with the other ring muscles of your body.

Contract, hold, release

Repeat this set five times.

Rest, and make sure that your breath is steady and free.

Repeat the same set ten times.

Bring your legs down and rest for a few minutes.

Bring your legs back up and now add your back sphincter to the routine as well, gently following your body's intuition.

Your mouth, eyes, nostrils, ears, and front and back sphincters are now contracting and releasing at the same time.

Repeat five times.

Rest.

Repeat ten times.

Release your legs to the ground and notice the chain reactions in your body. As before, these might include deep sighs, which indicate released tension, an urge to wiggle your toes, and a feeling of shifting alignments. Register these developments and do not force anything. Simply absorb this new awareness in your body.

When you feel that this realignment cycle has run its course, begin to conclude the session, following the same conclusion as you did in the previous session.

Rise from the floor with the least amount of effort. When you're standing on your feet, draw into your center and roll your head gently from side to side. When you feel centered and grounded, slowly move forward and rejoin your day.

The ring muscles exercise can be your solid foundation for health for your entire life. The contractions and releases of the ring muscles loosen the energy knots that your body routinely accumulates through the day. Doing these sets regularly helps to keep your body supple and responsive. Once the body restores its original equilibrium, it organically rallies to fight foreign invaders such as infections, cold, cuts, bruises, and more serious assaults to its immune system. The body knows how to do all this naturally; it was programmed to self-correct and self-repair—if we don't short-circuit its networks with bad habits and maintain it in good condition, from which it can function the way it was designed.

Touch Triggers

Touch triggers are psychosomatic devices for registering new awareness in your body in such a way that later you can recall this information at will. Touch triggers work by combining a psycho (mental) process with a somatic (physical) response to deposit a new memory at a specific point in your body, and later you'll be able to retrieve this useful information by touching that spot in your body.

As mentioned in the section on pressure points, your body retains memories of everything that we experience, good and bad. The unique benefit of the touch triggers is that they enable you to plant new awareness—new memories—in your body to create a permanent desirable change in our life.

The touch triggers can be any point of contact in your body. The most useful touch triggers are those that are easily accessible and that don't call much attention to themselves, such as pinching your earlobe, brushing the top of your head, or rubbing your thumb and forefinger together.

As we saw in Chapter 5, the mind controls the body. Thoughts—new information—create new forms. The distinctive feature of touch triggers is that they reinforce a physical experience with a mental process to register a new state of being in your body and mind.

Exercise: Touch Triggers

Relax and establish a free, effortless, steady pattern of breaths. Now think about a genuine problem that concerns you these days. It can be anything you're dealing with at the moment: a health issue, family dynamics, finances, or a challenging situation at work. Begin to rub your forefinger and thumb together while you tell yourself silently, "I am smart enough and strong enough, and I have the tools to solve this problem." Repeat this affirmation several times as you rub your forefinger and thumb, and pay attention to the sensation that this friction creates in your body. You can close your eyes at this point because it will help you to concentrate on the exercise. What you're doing here is planting in this spot an awareness that you can competently deal with this situation. This is all you need to do. Keep doing this for another minute as you repeat to yourself, "I am smart enough and strong enough, and I have the tools to solve this problem." Now we will slowly finish this exercise. This new awareness is now planted in that spot in your body.

Let's do another touch trigger exercise. We will deposit different information in another place in your body.

Using the tips of your forefinger and middle finger, gently rub the back of your other hand in a circular motion.

If you prefer, you can use just the tip of your forefinger, lightly pressing in the center of your hand. Breathe into the spot where your fingers touch the skin as you tell yourself silently, "Inhale freedom, exhale fear." Again say silently, "Inhale freedom, exhale fear." Simple as that. You can close your eyes, and keep rubbing the back of your hand, breathing into it and telling yourself silently, "Inhale freedom, exhale fear." Do this for another couple minutes. Now we'll finish this exercise. When you're ready, open your eyes and let's continue.

These touch triggers are so powerful because they're simple and easy to do. You've planted two pieces of useful information in your body, and you can recall them when you need that boost by touching those spots in your body. Part of the effectiveness of touch triggers is in how user-friendly they are. During your regular day you'll be able to repeat this sequence as many times as you like, because you can do it effortlessly as you go about your normal routines.

The more you do this exercise, the stronger this new awareness in your life will become. You can also deposit other information, with other affirmations, at other parts of your body.

Once I've mastered myself I've mastered the world.

CHAPTER TEN

Self-Management Skills

As noted previously, body consciousness techniques help us develop awareness of our body and trust in our intuition, which together lead to sensing in ourselves our optimal duration of existence. Yet, understanding how long we could reasonably live in our body is only the first part of the equation. The other crucial part is acquiring the self-management skills that would enable us to realize this potential. Self-management skills help you create the conditions in which you can live the longest and healthiest life possible in this given body.

Many important character traits go into making a successful life, among them creativity, discipline, faith, judgment, patience, and courage. However, the focus of this book is to help you identify in yourself your potential duration of existence and help you to be at your best condition at every age. Different individuals have different needs so there's no one-size-fits-all strategy. However, there are basic requirements that create the conditions in which we live our longest and healthiest life. This chapter covers the four essential self-management skills that lead to optimal lifespan and on which all the other useful qualities of life can be built.

The latest medical studies describe the relationship that genes and lifestyle choices play in determining a person's longevity as roughly 30 to 70 percent in favor of lifestyle choices.[1] As indicated in Chapter 5, the genetic blueprint we inherit is a potential, not a destiny. Family history is an important element in determining our approximate life span, but the crucial factor in affecting the quality and quantity of our life is our behavior. For example, the current U.S. life expectancy is an average of 79 years. However:

- Lifelong smoking causes coronary heart disease, lung cancer, and cancer of mouth, throat, bladder, and kidney; and can shorten life span by an average of ten years.
- Lifelong obesity causes cancer, heart disease, stroke, diabetes, kidney and liver diseases; and can cost you seven years.
- Chronic stress causes stroke, raises blood pressure and heart rate, and affects glucose levels, which regulate metabolism and balance in the body, all of which can shorten life span by eight years.
- Physical inactivity shuts down metabolism, and increases the risk of cardiovascular disease, diabetes, stroke, heart disease, breast cancer, and colon cancer; and can cost you nine years.
- Having fast food as your regular diet, full of calories from refined sugars and hydrogenated fats, very high in sodium, and very low in dietary fiber and essential vitamins and minerals, can shorten your life by ten years.
- A Canadian study published in October 2017 that followed thousands of adults over a period of fifty-nine years shows that long-term depression can shorten lifespan by an average of a decade or more.[2]

Just as we have seen in superstring theory that energy and matter are indivisible components of the central unit of existence, it is good to think of your mind and body as inseparable parts of your overall condition of wellbeing. They depend on each other and inform each other for the healthy operation of the entire unit that is you.

The greatest wisdom of existence sometimes consists in smallest choices: eat well, sleep well, treat yourself and others well.

Breathing

Breath is the foundation of everything, and everything begins with breath. Breath is the true barometer by which to measure your mental, physical, and emotional states: levels of anxiety, fitness, tightness, ease, or stress. The quality of your breath indicates how balanced and aligned the different systems of your body are at any given time.

The life force coursing through your body manifests itself through your breath.

We don't pay much attention to this activity and do it automatically about 22,000 times a day, but as the satirical publication *The Onion* correctly pointed out in October 2017, "A report released by the National Institutes of Health found that breathing can extend a person's lifespan by several decades. . . . Steady inhaling, when combined with equal parts exhaling, promotes healthy brain function. Conversely, missing even one day of breathing can drastically reduce an otherwise healthy person's life expectancy."[3]

We begin the self-management skills with breathing, because when we learn how to master our breath we can be in control in every situation in life. Our daily routines are filled with small and big annoyances, and potential causes of anxiety. When we find ourselves in a "tight situation," the natural tendency of the body is to stiffen, and the breath to become shallow or restricted. These are the hereditary responses of our survival mechanism: the fight, flight, or freeze instinct.

The solution for situations like these is to learn to do the opposite: breathe deeply and evenly. What you want to carry with you throughout life is the clear understanding that your breath is your personal domain, and no one can enter this private space uninvited. It is your castle, and the firm ground on which you can stand no matter how dangerous a certain situation might seem. Whatever negative circumstances we encounter, we can always draw inside, center ourselves, and regulate our breath—deep, steady, and free.

Here are some helpful mantras to carry in your mental toolkit and repeat silently to yourself when you face a tight situation:

- *My strength is in my breath.*
- *When I control my breath, I control my life.*
- *The oxygen of the whole world is available to me.*

This last idea is especially useful. Realize that you're never at a lack for oxygen. There's always plenty of air around you to fill your lungs to full capacity, so you never feel deprived of breath or anxious for space or safety. Following is a simple exercise which will help you develop mastery of your breath.

Note of caution: If you are pregnant, make sure that your condition allows you to do these deep breathing exercises.

Exercise: Mindful Breathing

The advantage of the following set is that it can be done anywhere and anytime, standing, sitting, walking, or lying on the floor. As you will see, you can also break it down to small segments, and do portions of it as you go about your daily activities.

Get comfortable and concentrate on your breath. Make sure it's steady, even, and free.

Now inhale on the count of 5.

Exhale without count.

Inhale again on the count of 5.

Exhale without count.

Repeat this sequence three times.

Now inhale without count, and exhale on the count of 5.

Repeat this sequence three times.

Now inhale on the count of 10. (It helps here to use your fingers as visual reminders, so you don't exert yourself mentally while focusing on your breath.)

Exhale without count.

Repeat this sequence three times.

Now inhale without count, and exhale on the count of 10.

Repeat this sequence three times.

Now slowly inhale on the count of 15, using your fingers to keep track. If counting to 15 proves too difficult, don't worry about it; you will gradually build up to it. Instead count to 12.

Exhale without count.

Repeat this sequence three times.

Now inhale without count, and exhale on the count of 15 or 12.

Repeat this sequence three times.

We will end this set now, and you can repeat it as many times as you like as you go about your daily routines.

The huge benefit of this little exercise is that it shows you that you are in control of your breath. The fact that you are able to pace your breath over the count of 5, and then 10, and then 12 or 15, is a clear sign that you have made your breath a conscious activity, which you can manage. It's no longer something that simply happens. You have now made it a deliberate event that you can monitor and regulate in every situation in your life.

Because you can master your breath in the contained environment of this exercise, the more you practice these sets, the more you'll be in charge of your breath in every circumstance you encounter. When you face a crisis of some kind that threatens to get out of control, you can center on your breath—because this is something that you *can* control—and let your breath carry you to safety.

Good Nutrition

The market is inundated with nutrition advice that is complicated, faddish, contradictory, and frightening people into believing that food is an enemy that needs to be controlled or avoided. In this section, we want to dispel any secrets regarding good nutrition, and to provide simple and sensible choices that will enable you to both enjoy food and manage your weight over a lifetime.

To put it plainly, what we eat becomes our body. Our body metabolizes (converts) what we eat into energy and nutrients, and there's a direct link between what we put in our body and the condition of the body. Our brain weighs only about 2 percent of our body mass but consumes roughly 20 percent of the oxygen and nutrients that we intake.[4]

Recent health statistics show that global obesity rates are rising steadily, with accompanying health problems that include severe joint pain, high blood pressure, diabetes, stroke, heart disease, high cholesterol, and sleep apnea. These increasing obesity trends are especially true in industrialized nations, such as the United States, United Kingdom, Australia, New Zealand, and Canada. But more and more countries are joining this undesirable club.

It's important to acknowledge from the start that it is very hard for most people to change their eating habits to lose weight and keep it off for the duration. The vast majority of diets are effective for just a short period of time because they're based on restricting our food consumption to only certain items. After a while, this causes our body and psyche to rebel. People react by binging, which creates the yo-yo effect—gaining a lot of weight, losing a lot of weight—and this is harmful to the body. The much better and longer-lasting approach is to learn the basic rules of good nutrition, and then to eat everything that you like in moderation. This way you won't feel that you're depriving yourself of foods you love, which is the downfall of every diet.

In general, you don't need complicated guidelines to provide good energy for your body. Keep it simple: Get most of your nutrients from vegetables, fruits, nuts, and lean protein such as poultry, fish, soya products, beans, and seeds; and satisfy all your cravings in a responsible manner.

Stay away from packed and processed foods as much as possible. Nothing that comes in a pill or a powder is better than what is found in nature. Avoid refined (white) sugar and white bread, and stay away from preservatives, chemical additives, and hydrogenated fats. These simple lifelong choices will ensure that you treat food not as something to be feared or avoided, but as a source of joy and of clean energy for your body. They will also assure that your weight never gets out of hand.

Rather than looking for nutrients and vitamins in processed supplements, it is better to obtain them as close as possible to nature, where these nutrients originate. This also requires a shift in our thinking from treating illnesses after they happen to healthy preventive habits, from playing catch-up to being proactive, and from deterring trouble before it occurs. In the spirit of making nutrition guidelines as simple as possible, just remember that it's better to get the vitamins from a fruit than a pill.

A key custom of residents in the Blue Zones—areas in the world with documented high percentages of centenarians (people aged one hundred and above) and super-centenarians (people aged 110 and above)—is that they seldom eat anything that comes wrapped in plastic.

Let's be real: If you live in Tulsa, Oklahoma, or Ocala, Florida, your environment is very different from that of Sardinia or Okinawa (two of the Blue Zones). Good nutritious food is not cheap and is not easily found everywhere. On the other hand, many people spend a lot more time on trivial activities than they do shopping for healthy food. What is more important to you? Do you consider nutrition a fast, thoughtless process in which you open the refrigerator, grab whatever's in there, stick it in the microwave, and wolf it down as you watch TV? This is your body and your home for this life. We determine the quality and quantity of our lifespan by the small choices we make in our daily routines.

All the different systems in our body (nervous, limbic, digestive, immune, respiratory, thyroid, skeletal, neurotransmitter, reproductive, endocrine) are connected to each other, and the operation of any one system affects all the others. This is an extra incentive to keep our body in good condition. As noted in Chapter 8, our body is naturally designed to regulate and heal itself if we don't harm it with bad habits and we keep it in adequate condition so it is able to do what it's been programmed to do.

Granted, finding fresh vegetables and fruits in the market may require a personal commitment, but this is an effort that pays for itself in the long run in health, wealth, and enjoyment of life. Here's the vicious cycle: People lose health to gain wealth, and then spend their hard-earned wealth to try to regain their health. However, because of the biological processes taking place in the body, these are conditions that can't be reversed. In most cases, the damage and neglect have gone on for so long, and the bad habits have been ingrained so deeply, that a significant improvement in overall wellness is no longer possible. The more effective approach is to see health as the true wealth and arrange our daily lives so we can be the best version of ourselves at every stage.

As you begin to develop good nutrition habits, it'll help you to always have handy your favorite fruits and nuts. If fresh fruit is not available, even small marketplaces carry packaged fruits. These are not as good as fresh produce but are still much better than processed snacks. Some people have never tasted dried fruits such as figs, dates, papaya, cherries, and mango. If you are one of these, try them; your body will really appreciate this. Fruits are nature's dessert and are packed with nutrients. Figs and dates and grapes and berries have been the preferred treats of royals for millennia. We give our bodies good, clean energy when we eat fruit on a regular basis.

When you are out and about, rather than purchasing a quick packaged snack out of a vending machine, carry with you a banana, an apple, a pear, or a bag of raisins to hold you over between meals. Once you have done this for some time, you will notice a remarkable difference in the clarity and operation of your body. Fruits are the equivalent of using the highest-octane gas in the tank of your Ferrari instead of filling your body with junk fuel.

Another good measure to go by is to have about 10 daily servings of fruits and vegetables. An important point to make here is that to maintain this as a lifelong habit, rather than a diet you do for several months and then revert to your old ways, find the fun in this new approach, and eat the fruits and vegetables you like—not because someone else told you, but because they are delicious, and you know you're treating your body to the best energy source there is. This is how we live our longest and healthiest life.

You can boil down good nutrition rules to a single catchy phrase: 70 percent fruits and vegetables, 30 percent whatever you want.

Proper Rest

Rest is a crucial component in your overall framework of wellness. Without proper rest the body and the mind cannot complete their natural cycles of cleansing, healing, and resetting, and cannot function adequately if sufficient relaxation periods are not provided.

Considering our modern 24/7 society, it is no surprise that recent studies find that a third of American adults are not getting enough sleep on a regular basis, and that this inadequate sleep has negative consequences both on personal and national levels. This has led the Center for Disease Control and Prevention (CDC) to declare insufficient sleep a "public health problem."[5]

Shortened sleep, which is less than seven to nine hours per night, has been shown to be a factor in about half of the leading causes of death in the United States, including accidents, hypertension, diabetes, and cardiovascular disease. And research conducted in 2016 by the non-profit group RAND Europe found that the U.S. economy loses up to $411 billion a year (2 percent of the GDP) due to insufficient sleep, which is an equivalent of roughly 1.2 million working days. Japanese economy, in second place in this study, loses up to $138 billion a year.[6]

Another sobering statistic is that a person sleeping on average less than six hours a night has a 10 percent higher mortality risk than someone sleeping between seven and nine hours.[7]

All living organisms on Earth have an internal biological clock of the circadian cycles, and these regulate your basic rhythms of digestion and elimination, heart rate, blood pressure, sleep patterns, body temperature, and balanced energy levels.

In October 2017, the Nobel Prize in Physiology or Medicine was awarded to Jeffrey Hall, Michael Rosbash, and Michael Young for helping to explain how plants, animals, and humans adapt their biological rhythm so that it is synchronized with the Earth's revolutions. The Nobel committee noted that "with exquisite precision, our inner clock adapts our physiology to the dramatically different phases of the day. The clock regulates critical functions such as behavior, hormone levels, sleep, body temperature, and metabolism."[8]

In order to have optimal health, our brain and body require a steady 24-hour rhythm. In today's world that is open for business around the clock, if we try to defy our circadian rhythms we will inevitably come up against the biological limits of our internal clocks. The body's well-being is affected when there is a misalignment between our internal biological clock and the external environment. When there's imbalance between our lifestyle and our inner clock, this affects the body's metabolism and hormone regulation, and can lead to a number of diseases, such as diabetes, cancer, and Alzheimer's.

A clear example of our inner clock being out of sync with Earth's clock is experiencing jet lag after traveling across multiple time zones. As noted, each of us has an internal biological clock that regulates our circadian rhythms. This internal master clock is in sync with the external 24-hour cycle of day and night because it gets its cues from light exposure. When we jump over multiple time zones fast with jet travel, this leaves our inner clock lagging behind the outer clock, which means that our circadian rhythms get out of sync with our current physical location. Depending on the number of time zones skipped, it can take us a few days to recover from feeling groggy, being in a haze, spikes or drops in appetite, and a general state of being off-center. Jet lag is an interruption of our body's regular rhythms.

Here as well, we can see an analogy between the finite amount of energy that our body contains, and the finite amount of time in a 24-hour day and night cycle. These are both frameworks that need to be respected and adapted to if we are to live a healthy and long life.

The deepest meditation that you can undergo occurs during sleep. It is during sleep that the brain arranges the mental furniture it has accumulated through the day, gets rid of unnecessary debris, files away information in the subconscious for later use, and cleanses and prepares for the following day. This is also what is meant by getting out of the body's way and allowing it to restore its equilibrium.

The human brain is an electrochemical organ, and normal brain activity sends out signals in the form of frequency waves at different ranges. There are five levels of frequency range: gamma, beta, alpha, theta, and delta. The following chart lists the different states of brain activity, from the highest level of peak performance down to the lowest level of deep sleep, and describes the important role that each state plays in our overall health.

Brainwave Frequencies

30 > 100 Hz	Gamma waves	Gamma waves are a recent discovery that resulted from the development of digital electroencephalography (EEG) machines. Earlier analog EEG recorders could not read brainwaves at those high frequencies. Gamma frequencies are associated with heightened self-awareness and insight, and are found commonly in long-term practitioners of meditation. Gamma waves denote a state of peak mental and physical performance, when the senses are extraordinarily sharp, at exceptional circumstances such as walking on a wire or "being in the zone" at an athletic or artistic event. Gamma waves also connote greater lucidity of thought and improved intuition.
12 > 30 Hz	Beta waves	Beta frequencies are associated with being fully awake, concentration, thinking, alertness, being focused, or being engaged in any form of activity, such as reading this sentence. This is the state in which most people are during the day.

8 > 12 Hz	Alpha waves	Alpha brainwaves occur when a person is relaxed or begins to get drowsy but is still awake and conscious. This is the state between sleep and wakefulness, and during this state a person is awake but resting.
		Alpha brain patterns are divided into deep alpha, a state of deep relaxation (twilight state between sleep and waking), and higher alpha, a more focused but still a relaxed state.
		The brain in alpha wave patterns is very absorbent to stimuli and is receptive for programming the subconscious, effective learning of new material, and self-hypnosis.
		This state is also conducive to high levels of creativity and expression.
4 > 8 Hz	Theta waves	Theta state is best known as the state in which rapid eye movement (REM) sleep occurs. It is the state of being asleep, dreaming, and even deep and effective meditation.
		The brain in theta state produces a number of significant benefits, among them enhanced long-term memory, better immune system, sustained attention over time, increased creativity and receptivity to new ideas, as well as more acute problem-solving.
		As part of the body's built-in correction mechanism, when the brain slows down to the lower patterns of theta state, it produces relaxing endorphins that organically melt the body's stress away.

0.5 > 4 Hz	Delta waves	Delta waves occur when we are in a deep sleep and are known for triggering the release of human growth hormone (HGH), which is the body's natural way of repairing itself. This is why long hours of sleep are beneficial when recovering from injury or illness.
		Delta waves are also associated with very deep states of meditation. At the delta level the body regenerates its energy, relieves stress, and revives the immune system. The delta state reinvigorates our mind, body, and spirit. When a person's predominant brainwave is delta, the body is restoring itself and resetting its internal clocks.

In the course of a typical day we experience a combination of all the different frequencies in the chart, but according to the task we are performing at the moment we will manifest a particular frequency over others.

As we age, diminished quantities of human growth hormone in our body manifest in various forms, such as decreased muscle tone, increased weight gain, loss of stamina, wrinkled skin lacking good tone and texture, and reduced memory capacity. Human growth hormone is produced naturally by the pituitary gland, which is situated in the center of our brain. When a person is in deep and dreamless sleep at the delta brainwave level the pituitary gland is stimulated to produce more HGH, which is why we feel refreshed and replenished after a good night's sleep.

Think of deep sleep as preventive medicine: Relaxation at the delta level releases the human growth hormone, which stimulates the anti-aging properties that the body uses to revitalize itself. An overall framework of a healthy diet, balanced lifestyle, and a calm mental and emotional state also helps the body to generate HGH.

How to get more quality sleep? Here are some ideas:

- Keep regular hours for going to bed and waking up, so your body can develop a familiar rhythm.
- Make your environment conducive to falling asleep. This means to eliminate noise and make your room as dark as possible.
- Avoid caffeine and alcohol close to bedtime.
- Drink herbal, non-caffeinated tea, such as chamomile tea. Chamomile is known to help you fall asleep.
- To help your digestive system, have your last meal at least two hours before bedtime.
- Read a good book or an article. This will help you to put the day behind you and naturally transition to sleep.
- Other things that can help you improve your sleep are avoiding smoking and getting regular physical activity, and before bedtime using relaxation techniques such as yoga and meditation.

Listen to the flow of life inside you; listen to the force of life inside you. Listen to the rhythm of your body; listen to the rhythm of the world.

Active Lifestyle

In this chapter I want to show in plain and simple terms that making healthy choices in one's life is fun and with smart planning can be fit into our daily routines. Not only is this not difficult, but the other way around. Neglecting our body through sedentary habits, inactivity, and inattention leads to a condition in which we feel sluggish, drained, and fatigued. Conversely, simple, sound habits such as good nutritious food, regular physical activity, and balanced lifestyle lead to a sense of vitality, energy, strength, and the confidence that we are living our best possible life.

The human body needs exercise to help the bones, muscles, and heart function optimally, but people are less and less active as they spend more and more time in cars and in front of computers. A study published in the medical journal *Lancet* in July 2012 shows that inactivity is a risk factor in mortality comparable to smoking or obesity. The three leading causes of premature death at this time are tobacco, poor diet, and lack of physical activity.[9]

Inactivity leads to being out of shape, which leads to illnesses and diseases, because the body's natural recuperating processes have been thwarted by being unfit, which further perpetuates this vicious cycle—because the body is not in good condition it is more susceptible to harm, and because of this poor shape it cannot fight these illnesses effectively. On the other hand, a healthy body regularly wards off sicknesses before they occur and, when they do occur, fights them more readily. It is not that healthy people don't get sick, but when they do, because the body is able to operate as it was designed, they bounce back into full health a lot quicker.

Exercise is a major factor in reducing diabetes and other diseases because by strengthening your muscles and providing a steady supply of oxygen to your lungs and heart, you boost your immune system and keep the body in a condition in which it can stay healthy, as it is naturally programmed to do.

As long as the human body is made of flesh, blood, and bones, what was true for first humans will remain true for us: Health is the true wealth.

Remember that the brain is part of the body. Activities that are good for your body can also sharpen your brain: Physical exercise improves neurogenesis, the continuous growth of nerve cells in the brain, which further boosts the immune system. This is a process that you can help maintain well into your higher decades—by keeping both the body and the mind fit.

Physical activity is essential to our mental and physical health because the mind is based in the brain, and the brain, as mentioned, requires 20 percent of the oxygen and nutrients that we intake.

How does exercise improve the functioning of mind and body? Physical activity causes the body to produce chemicals called endorphins.

Endorphins are natural narcotics that the body makes to reduce the perception of pain, and that can make us feel euphoric. That's how after steady exercise we reach the "runner's high," an overall feeling of well-being and balance in the body. This in turn reduces mental stress and boosts our self-esteem, with the knowledge that we are in charge of our own wellness and doing what makes us feel at our best.

Let's now demystify physical activity. No one expects us to become Olympic athletes. Rather, we are talking about simple and sensible activities that can easily fit into our daily routines:

- Walking for thirty minutes several times a week.
- Taking the stairs instead of the elevator when it makes sense.
- Walking manageable distances instead of jumping in a car out of habit just to go a few blocks.
- Riding a bicycle.
- Getting up and stretching on a lunch break to generate better blood flow in your body.
- Hiking on weekends.
- Arranging your lifestyle to where you can be as active as possible during your normal day.

Some people have the misconception of exercise as being all or nothing, that if they don't make it to the gym several times a week, they've fallen off the wagon. That is both wrong and self-defeating. A much better approach is that something is better than nothing. Small adjustments in everyday life lead to a lifetime of wellness.

Seen clearly, fitness doesn't mean a bulked-up, muscle-bound man who spends hours in the gym pumping iron, or an over-exercised, over-worked woman who has no time to relax, but true balanced lifestyle consists of understanding that the human body needs physical activity to stay healthy, and incorporating practical, sustainable, and comfortable choices into our daily routines.

A helpful mantra: Sweat cleanses places water can never reach.

Staying Fit in Higher Decades

So far we have focused on physical health span. Now let's review mental health span and how to stay vibrant as we grow in age. As we saw in Chapter 4 on the brain's plasticity, neurogenesis means the growth of new cells, and contrary to previous dogma, studies have shown that the brain produces new neurons until the day we die. This simply means that the brain is capable of learning new things as long we are alive.[10]

One of the key features that emerged from these new understandings of neuroplasticity is the principle of "use it or lose it." Like any other muscle that weakens from inactivity, if we don't exercise the cells in our brains they atrophy and die.

To stay vital and brain-healthy into our higher decades, the key is to take up activities that stimulate both our body and mind, and utilize different aspects of our being: mental, physical, and emotional. The more complex the task, the more synapses (new connections) are generated in your brain. Make this activity as challenging as possible, but not too challenging so it becomes a chore. You want to maintain a sense of fun and novelty. The best activities to keep both our minds and bodies engaged in higher decades are:

- Learning a new language—far from your native tongue. That means a different family of languages, with an unfamiliar alphabet and uncommon pronunciations. For example, if your first language is English, try tackling Chinese, Japanese, Urdu, or Arabic. But if these languages don't appeal to you, no worries: Even learning French or German will stimulate new regions in your brain.
- Learning a new dance. Dance stimulates your mental and motor skills, with the added benefit of a social interaction that is a boost for longevity.
- Travel to new places to absorb different culture, pace, food, and customs.

- Learning a new musical instrument.
- Playing challenging board games.
- Staying socially engaged with friends and family. This contributes to a longer and healthier life because it provides us with accountability for our attitude and actions, gives us a safety net we can depend on in emergencies, and generally adds flavor and meaning to our life in knowing we are loved and valued.

These activities are helpful to keep your mind and body in great shape because they require intense focus. Concentration is a key part in brain health because it means that the brain is fully engaged. All these activities use different aspects of our being, such as motor skills, mental skills, and mind-body coordination. This is also a very good way to prevent depression and weight gain, and to ward off diseases such as Alzheimer's and dementia.

In *The Brain that Changes Itself,* Norman Doidge quotes Michael Merzenich, whose pioneering research starting at the end of the twentieth century laid down the foundations for the science of neuroplasticity, as saying, "Everything that you can see happen in a young brain can happen in an older brain. The only requirement is that the person must have enough of the reward, or punishment, to keep paying attention through what might otherwise be a boring training session." If so, Merzenich says, "the changes can be every bit as great as the changes in a newborn."[11]

Life is a special gift that's best experienced with a sense of joy and meaning. The guidelines listed in this chapter are not a straitjacket to hem us into a restricted life but a sensible framework for our entire life span. If you crave an occasional indulgence—steak, cake, an alcoholic beverage you love, or anything else—the smart thing to do is satisfy that desire, knowing that afterward you'll bounce back into the healthy overall structure that the principles in this chapter provide.

This is the state called rejuvenation: the body's innate ability to restore itself to good health, and no one can give this to you but you.

PART FOUR

Everyday Applications

You are an individual human expression of infinite cosmic potential. Anything you can conceive you can create.

CHAPTER ELEVEN

Mental Imagery Tools

This part of the book lists a baker's dozen of mental imagery tools that can be used for dealing skillfully with life's different situations. The subconscious mind processes information not in terms of words and numbers but in terms of images and pictures. Mental imagery techniques are effective communication channels to the body's autonomic nervous system, the part of the neural network that regulates basic functions, such as heart rate, blood pressure, and digestion. In this way, mental imagery tools help you to manage your passage through life in a competent manner, while at the same time contributing to your body's harmonious operation. In other words, they help you align the world inside you with the world outside.

You may find that certain aspects of the individual mental tools listed here "spill" into each other and color each other. This is normal for mental imagery techniques, because by their nature they are flexible and fluid. This characteristic of mental imagery adds an additional benefit for you as it trains your mind to think creatively and without restrictions.

The distinguishing traits of creativity are flexibility of perception, a willingness to experience new things, a highly developed sense of intuition, tolerance of ambiguity, psychological risk-taking, independent thought and judgment, and the ability to see structure in chaos. It is quite obvious that not only creative types, but every person can benefit by developing these traits for an enjoyable and successful journey through life.

When you approach these mental imagery sequences for the first time, it'll help you to use the meditation techniques (refer to Chapter 9) to get centered and focused.

Obey the laws of nature and follow your imagination.

Visualization

Overview

Visualization is a highly effective sensory instrument that is used as a foundation for many different imagery techniques. Every mental imagery tool listed in this part of the book contains in it aspects of visualization. It helps to remember that the words *imagery* and *imagining* are synonyms for *visualization*.

Visualization employs the conceptual powers of the mind to create mental pictures of situations, places, tasks, memories, feelings, or anything else you would like to access through your senses and your imagination.

There are two kinds of visualization: past and future. Past is called "sense memory," because it relies mainly on our bodily senses to recall a past event in the most vivid pictures; and future is called simply "visualization," because it primarily uses powers of imagining to establish in our mind a clear vision of an event that we would like to become real.

When applying the visualization method, both past and future, be as specific and concrete as you can, and use as many of your senses as possible: smell, hearing, vision, touch, and taste. This will draw a sharp and three-dimensional picture of the experience you want to create.

When you draw a clear image of an event that you want to materialize in life, you are creating a multidimensional and multisensory engagement that includes your mind, body, intention, and imagination, and sets into motion a whole series of little steps that lead to the picture you have created. To be clear, this doesn't mean that that image will simply pop up into the broad light one day; it means that you have now put into action a mental, physical, and fully conscious campaign. You have initiated the chain reaction that has the potential to result in the outcome you've imagined.

Outstanding athletes rehearse this mental practice systematically as part of their conditioning. In a one-hundred-meter dash a runner in the blocks visualizes the gun going off, and her taking off from the blocks at just the right angle and with the focus that she had practiced over and over in training sessions. She sees herself achieving her full speed at approximately forty meters. She is prepared to use every ounce of energy and breath in her body, and she imagines herself crossing the finish line by thrusting forward her upper body.

Visualization is such a potent tool for mastery and performance because as far as neuroscience is concerned there is little difference between imagining an act and actually doing it. Brain scans show that acting or imagining activates the same motor and sensory processes in the brain. By rehearsing in our mind the sequence of events that we want to put in motion, we prime the area in the brain that is responsible for that activity, so it's ready to repeat the same steps when we actually take the action.[1]

Applications of Past: Sense Memory

You would want to recall a sense memory of an event that you've experienced in the past to help put yourself in the right frame of mind and prepare you for a present challenge. For example, if you are going on a job interview tomorrow, it will help you to evoke a memory of a past event in which you were at your optimal condition: smart, competent, and successful. This state of being will ensure that you show up to the meeting tomorrow at the best shape that you can be.

Another example would be if you are beginning to date a new person and want to handle this initial phase with just the right mixture of mastery, elegance, confidence, and cool. In this case, you would want to recall a past relationship or a past situation in which you felt appreciated for simply being who you are, without having to push anything and without feeling needy.

The way memory-retrieval mechanism works is that by recalling various specific details of that experience you unlock a whole network of associations related to that event. This creates a sharp image of that past experience in your mind and makes it possible to project that past feeling on to future events. There is no difference, as far as the visual cortex is concerned, between seeing a red rose and imagining it. The essence of red is present in both.

The System for Past: Sense Memory

Make yourself comfortable, relax, and concentrate on your breath. Make sure it is steady, deep, and free. Let's use the example of you wanting to prepare yourself for an important appointment tomorrow, such as a job interview, by recalling from your past an experience in which you felt at your absolute best. (Once you become proficient with these exercises, you will be able to do them with your eyes closed, which will help you to focus your mind on the images you are creating.)

Run through the memory bank of your past experiences and see where you felt exactly how you want to be tomorrow. Don't belabor this process; don't overthink it. Trust your instincts. The first appropriate analogous event that comes to the forefront is most likely the right incident.

Now grow quiet, and revisit this past episode in your mind. The more specific details you will be able to recall the better you will be able to use this tool:

- What day of the week is this?
- Are you at home, outdoors, in what city, and so on?
- What time of the day is it?
- Are you alone or with company?
- What are you wearing?
- Is it spring, summer, or fall?

- What events led to this particular point where you feel at your optimal condition?

Recollect exactly what you did to create this great feeling:

- How did you earn this?
- What challenges, if any, did you have to overcome?
- What happens after this event?

Now, register in your mind and body precisely what you feel: appreciated, competent, accomplished, or proud of yourself.

Relax into this moment and take it all in. Absorb this potent and wonderful sensation in your body.

Now add a touch trigger (see Chapter 9), such as rubbing your thumb and forefinger together, or rubbing your earlobe, to the specific emotion you're experiencing at this moment. You will deposit this useful memory of being in your best shape at that past event at this particular place in your body (for example, thumb and forefinger, your earlobe, or any other convenient location) that you'll be able to access easily tomorrow as you prepare for your interview, or as you sit in the chair just before the appointment, ready to go in.

This is all there is to it. You have recalled a personal event at which you were at your best, you brought it forward in your mind, you made it available for future use, and you've planted it in a readily accessible spot in your body where you'll be able to use it any time you like.

Applications for Future: Visualization

In this set, you'll want to form a clear picture in your mind of something that you want to happen in the future. This can be any reasonable thing at all that conforms to the laws of nature—meaning no senseless imaginings like "I want to walk on Mars" or "I want to have a million bucks deposited in my bank account," if you're not willing to do the work that this vision would require.

As we have seen previously on these pages, anything that respects the fundamental laws of nature can be brought into reality. That possible eventuality is currently vibrating as a unit of potential amongst the myriad other probabilities floating in the ether of existence. You are currently the only person who sees this picture in your mind. Your job, as the person who wants to freeze this potential into existence, is to initiate a chain of activities that will result in the slice of reality that everyone else will be able to see and experience.

Imagination and action inform each other in many different ways, because the quicker you can imagine something the faster you can do it.

The System for Future: Visualization

As with the method that you used to recall the favorable past episode, the more details you are able to fill into this vision, the better chances you'll have of witnessing it in reality.

You need to recall that experience vividly to make it available for future use.

Relax; establish steady, deep, and effortless breaths; and concentrate on the situation that you want to create. Let's say you want to be promoted to the corner office at your firm. You want to be the boss (of your department or your regional division).

Paint a clear picture in your mind:

- Where is this corner office located? On what floor? How big is it? Is there sunlight coming in? Does it have bright fluorescent lights, or more subdued lighting?
- Do you get this office already furnished, or do you get to choose what desks, chairs, shelves, and computers you will use?
- Is there just one desk or several?
- Are you going to have a secretary, an assistant, or a deputy in your new position?

- What exactly are your responsibilities in this new position and how much time are you going to spend at work?
- How much are you getting paid?
- Where do you live when you have this job?
- What distance do you travel between home and work?
- Do you have a family at this point in your life?
- How many kids do you have, if any?
- Do you have pets?

Why do you want this vision to come about? This is not to pass moral judgment on your wish, but the fuller presence you are able to create of this future event in your imagination, the more chances you'll have to see it materialize in real life.

To increase traction for this vision in reality, think of it as both a physical and a mental practice. This means to see yourself, hear yourself, and feel yourself being in this new position, attending to your responsibilities in a competent manner, and being respected by your staff, and appreciated by your superiors.

Benefits of Past Sense Memory

- Increased self-knowledge and self-reliance: knowing that you have the tools inside you to bring yourself to a position where you can face any challenge in the best possible manner.
- Developing creativity and spatial thinking.
- Rich inner life, in which you realize the vast resources stored in your mental bank.

Benefits of Future Visualization

- Setting clear goals in mind, which is critical for focusing and harnessing your energies onto specific tasks.

- Knowing that you can accomplish what you set your heart and mind to do.
- Feeling in charge of your own destiny in life.

Fork in the Road

Overview

Every so often in life we come to a proverbial fork in the road and we need to decide which course to follow. The purpose of this exercise is to select the best option available to you at this juncture by seeing as far as possible down the different paths you are facing.

Applications

This old metaphor of a crossroads is a useful mental exercise to improve your judgment and boost your forward-planning skills. It is best applied in a situation that requires a sober assessment of different alternatives, and helps you to develop your sense of foresight, as well as your sense of authority to select the best option presented at the time and then stick to your decision.

The System

You are facing the symbolic fork in the road of several paths that lead down different directions and different outcomes. Your dilemma is which one to take.

Your first order of business is to narrow your choices to a manageable number of no more than four paths. This means that you select the most viable routes, with the least potential harm and with the greatest likelihood to generate your desired outcome.

In this initial winnowing-down process, you've made your first important decisions.

Now look down each trail that you've chosen as far as your eyes can see. Use your imagination to visualize conceivable opportunities, risks, and consequences.

To be clear, this is a lengthy process that requires attention, time, and effort, but the results will also be equal to the energy you invest to make the best selection.

Compile *all* existing information regarding the different options each path provides, and the likely outcomes they will generate.

Make the best decision at this juncture and stand behind this decision, knowing that this is the most educated choice you could make according to the data available at present.

Even if later your decision does not produce the desired outcome, even if it "proves to be wrong," it does not change the fact that at this point it was the best decision you could have made.

This is how we face life's tests head-on in the best fashion and grow into mature individuals able to make choices and then be accountable for our decisions.

Benefits

- Requires that you develop your vision of the outside conditions and insight into your inner responses, as you weigh the options that life presents you and how they resonate with your authentic needs.
- Improves your sense of prudence and level-headedness as you realize that every action that you take generates an appropriate chain reaction.
- Increases your confidence in your abilities to deal skillfully with life's different situations and handle yourself in a responsible manner.
- Teaches you to evaluate different alternatives while considering various simultaneous, interdependent factors that form the regular fabric of life.

Jigsaw Puzzle of Life

Overview

Just as in a jigsaw puzzle there are pieces of varying shapes, sizes, and colors that need to fit together snugly, so your larger picture of life also contains events, decisions, relationships, and arrangements that must fit together smoothly for your entire passage through existence to make perfect sense.

Applications

This image is best used to assess adding a new item into your overall framework of life, whether it's a relationship, buying a house, moving to a new city, or changing professions.

The System

This new ingredient under consideration needs to fit into the picture of your life without damaging, bending, scratching, or covering the other pieces on your canvas.

If you are weighing whether to join a new gym or a new club, you would consider several factors: the distance from your home, the type of membership that this club or gym attracts, their operating hours and whether this would fit with your daily and weekly routines, how joining this club would affect the other obligations in your life, and so forth.

Benefits

- Gives you a sense of proportion, and helps you develop a wider perception of how different events and elements of your existence might affect, enhance, or detract from each other.

- Sharpens your ability to see the larger perspective, which helps you to feel grounded in the present moment while maintaining a clear image of your entire passage through life.
- Improves your ability to make conscious decisions about your circumstances, which in turn increases your self-awareness and overall mastery of life.

Captain of the Ship

Overview

In this mental depiction, your journey through life is a ship, and you are the captain in charge of steering it to its destination. Your passengers are the people in your life to whom you are accountable: your spouse, your children, your parents, the employees of your company, or the members of your softball team.

Applications

Just like the open waters, the ocean of your life can hit rough weather, and it is up to you as the captain of your ship of life to guide it masterfully among the figurative shoals, icebergs, jutting rocks, and shallow passages. You need to avoid sudden maneuvers, to not inconvenience your passengers needlessly, and also to not take any other unnecessary risks that would endanger the lives of everyone who is dependent on your judgment.

The System

You are at the helm of your ship, piloting it to its destination. It is your responsibility to know the forecast, the route you'll be traveling, at what speed, the number of passengers on board, the inventory of supplies, and the overall condition of your vessel.

It is also your job to lay out the fastest, safest, and most beautiful itinerary to your target port.

If you are in charge of a crew of sailors, you need to know each person's strong and weak points, and how you'd be able to rely on each of them in case of an emergency.

Benefits

- Develops in you a sense of patience, prudence, overall perspective, and accountability for your actions.
- Improves your ability to think in detail and plan ahead.
- Deepens your sense of confidence, maturity, and leadership skills.

Hourglass

Overview

Each person is an hourglass of potential, into whom a variety of skills, talents, attributes, and character traits have been poured in different proportions, making them distinct individuals. You are a singular drop in the ocean of life, and also a part of the whole, just as a single drop of water is a representative part of the ocean, and the particular nature of the entire ocean is present in that single drop.

Your life at present is an hourglass in time. You are the sum total of the choices you've made in your life so far. The person you are today is a result of every action you have taken and avoided taking up to this point, and what you will be five and ten and thirty years from now will be a direct outcome of the thoughts you will think and the actions you will take from this moment on.

Applications

This mental routine is designed to give you a clear view of your present place in the universe, and the nature of the cosmic forces coursing through your body. You are an organic part of the world, and the powers that regulate the celestial bodies in space also influence the celestial body that is you.

The System

Grow quiet, establish steady and free breaths, and consider the fact that the spirit animating you is timeless. It enters your body when you are born, drives you for the length of your physical existence, and then it rejoins the eternal source.

Think of the fact that at this point in evolution you contain in your genes everything that the world has learned so far. The person that you are, here and now, is a result of cosmic, chemical, biological, and developmental processes that have been taking place in the universe for 13.7 billion years since the big bang. This is the nature of information, wisdom, and understanding that you carry in your genetic makeup.

From the perspective of an hourglass, this is the past that has resulted in the present that the specific person that is you is experiencing at this moment.

That past has resulted in this present. Your genetic evolutionary makeup also contains the possibilities of all imaginable futures: everything that conforms to the laws governing existence in the cosmos.

Everything that will happen in your life from this point on will be an outcome of the thoughts you'll have, the intentions that these thoughts will generate, where you will choose to apply your attention, and the actions that will derive from these factors. It is your privilege and responsibility to decide what experience you will have in life.

Benefits

- Gives you a strong grounding in the present moment against the backdrop of your larger passage through existence.
- Enables you to grasp the causal relation of the different events in your life.
- Helps you to see that the character of your entire journey consists in single, minute choices that you make on a daily basis.

This moment is an hourglass in eternity, sifting through one grain at a time, one thought at a time, one action at a time: the past passing into the future through the present.

Train Ride

Overview

This sequence helps you master whatever project you are currently working on by setting in place intermediary "train stations" that divide the entire big job into small manageable sections. You break down the large task into little portions along the road, and you shift your focus away from the massive task to the individual segments along the journey.

Applications

This undertaking can be any activity in which you are presently engaged (for example, training for a marathon, working on a doctorate, saving a certain amount of money, or losing weight).

You have broken down the huge task into small convenient parts, and you work on each part separately. When you arrive at the next station, you look back and register the progress, and this 1) gives you a sense of accomplishment; 2) keeps you from feeling overwhelmed by the enormity of the entire task; and 3) gives you a clear vision of your progress, which boosts your sense of confidence.

These intermediary train stations are your *visible goals*, attainable destinations within your reach—which you can see with your naked eyes. Every time you reach one of these goals, this gets you farther away from where you've come and closer still to where you're going, which further reassures you that you can cover the entire distance.

The System

See clearly in your mind your current stage in the project on which you are working.

Define precisely what the end destination of this project is.

Now divide the long path ahead of you into small logical sections.

Let's say you are training for your first marathon. The longest distance you've run now has been six miles.

You set for yourself the first station on your new train ride to be an eight-mile run. You gradually increase your running distance to reach eight miles, and when you do, you rest and acknowledge this accomplishment, because it gives you a sense of confidence that you can swing forward to your next challenge.

You set your next train station to be at the ten-mile mark. When you arrive there, look back, acknowledge the progress, and assimilate this new mental phase in your life.

You had never run a ten-mile distance before. See the distance you have already traveled, and this will further give you a boost that in this manner—of small, incremental parts—you can travel very far.

Depending on how much time you have before the actual marathon, set your next station to the fifteen-mile mark. You rest, look back, and again acknowledge your progress.

You set your next train station at the twenty-mile mark. When you arrive here, you see that the twenty-six-mile mark of the full marathon is within a striking distance.

You continue following this plan until you've run the full twenty-six miles. You can be proud of yourself. You've made this happen.

Benefits

- Helps you be more detail-oriented and accurate in your thinking.
- Develops your skills for logical and methodical planning.
- Gives you a well-deserved sense of confidence by knowing that you are in charge of the manner and rate of your progress.

This gives you a calm sense of mastery that you are in control of your instrument of mind-body-energy, and can create the conditions where you are at your best at every stage of your train ride through life.

Radio Beacon

Overview

This imagery tool is most helpful when you are working on a specific goal and want the shortest, most effective, and most elegant way to reach that target. In this sequence, you place the accomplishment of your goal—a radio beacon that emits constant signals—at your desired destination, and you adjust your progress toward this goal according to the strength of the signals that you receive.

The broadcasting tower located at the conclusion of your goal is emitting radio signals in all directions. You have a receiver inside you, and just as with radio reception when you drive through the mountains, sometimes the reception is clear and sometimes it isn't. In your daily circumstances, this faulty reception can translate into any number of obstructions: You feel out of sorts, sleepy, sluggish, distracted, or generally unable to concentrate on what you know you need to do to move toward your target.

Applications

Your job is to get the clearest reception in your body and mind of the signals coming from the radio tower. This might mean stepping away from whatever you're doing right now to simply go and have a big juicy steak, have a piece of fruit, watch a movie, go for a run, or take a nap. You need to trust yourself and trust your body. This exercise is a perfect means for you to tune into the messages that your body is sending you on a regular basis. Does it feel hungry, tired, thirsty, sleep-deprived, or overworked? These routines are how you come to identify the natural rhythm of your body and recognize your body's needs. You have to trust these processes and allow them the time to complete their cycles. This is how you develop your body's intuition and learn to create the conditions in which you can be at your best mentally, physically, and emotionally at every point in your life.

The System

The radio beacon technique is useful to make a decision that requires foresight, focus, clarity, and simultaneous assessment of several objects at once.

Let's say that you're planning to move to a new city or a new country, but you are not sure when the best time to make the transition is, whether you are ready for this move or not, and whether you should sell your house and belongings in this city or country and start from fresh in the new location. The alternative would be to keep your current home in this city as a safety net on which you could fall back if things in the new location don't work out as you plan.

Use here the general guidelines of meditation exercises in Chapter 9. Make yourself comfortable, grow quiet, and establish a free, effortless, steady pattern of breaths.

Place the radio beacon at the exact center of the future you envision in the new location. If you are going there to start a new job, include this new job as part of the full picture of reality you are creating in your mind. Include also a new comfortable house, a car if you are planning on getting one, a circle of friends, a professional network, and any other detail that will make your life satisfactory, healthy, enjoyable, and balanced.

If you are going there for a relationship, build the mental picture of your desired situation around this factor. The radio signal should have in it every important ingredient of the reality you create.

Draw inside you and access your center; this is where your inner receiver is located. Whether you use here a meditation routine or any other favorite activity, such as taking a walk, swimming, or going for a bike ride, it is essential to adjust your receiver to the position that gets the clearest signal from the broadcasting tower at your destination.

Think in terms of dangling your receiver this way or that, or moving it up or down, right or left, just as you would to improve the reception on your mobile phone.

Because life can be complex and contain many unforeseeable obstacles, this fine-tuning process might be challenging and time-consuming. You develop confidence in your own instincts by recognizing when the reception is sufficiently clear for you to make a decision, or when an approaching deadline requires that you make the best decision possible at this point. In this circumstance, you register the strongest signals that you're receiving from your body, heart, and mind, and you follow them with a set of practical actions that will lead you in the most direct manner toward your desired destination. Mastery of yourself and your inner resources consists in this simple and confident approach.

Benefits

- Teaches you to prioritize your actions.
- Sharpens your instincts and focuses your vision for a prudent conduct in life.

- Improves your self-knowledge and self-confidence in realizing that you can make serious choices in your life in an educated manner, and then accept responsibility for these actions and stand behind them with full authority and commitment.

Tightrope

Overview

This mental imagery technique applies to a situation or an undertaking where the boundaries are well-defined, and the manner of execution is strictly prescribed. This figurative tightrope can connect two remote events, locations, or mental states of being, and the walk that a person does on this tightrope can likewise last different lengths of time or distance.

The documentary *Man on Wire* describes how Philippe Petit walked above the 110th floors between the Twin Towers in New York City on August 6, 1974. He and his crew rigged a wire between the two buildings overnight, and in the morning Petit got on the tightrope and spent the following forty-five minutes walking between the towers back and forth. As the cameras recorded, midway between the buildings he lay down on the five-eighths-of-an-inch-thick wire and rested on his back for several minutes with total composure and peace. Witnesses who were interviewed afterward by TV stations described what they had seen as profound and sublime.

Applications

The popular image of a tightrope is often used metaphorically in various realms of life, such as politics, as in "walking the diplomatic tightrope between the clashing interests of his diverse constituents"; the arts, as in "an artist's life is a tightrope walk"; or sports, as in "walking the tightrope of expectations of his teammates and fans." The essential elements at play during a tightrope walk are precision, balance, focus, and relaxation.

Sometimes a tightrope stretches over a finite length of time or distance, and you can manage your energy and behavior accordingly (as, for example, in the train ride imagery). At other times, we can't quite know how long this tightrope walk might last. In this scenario, once we have walked on this tightrope for a while, we discover that *the secret of mastering a tightrope walk is in learning to relax on it.*

Rather than "holding our breath" in anticipation of arriving finally at our destination to be able to relax, the only viable way to survive on this open-ended tightrope walk is by making ourselves comfortable—*right here and now.*

By extension, this is what living our longest and healthiest life really means. We learn how to create the best conditions in our lives, regardless of outside circumstances, here and now. A basic formula for this is: Eat well, sleep well, and treat yourself and others well. Be a good animal and listen to your body. Your body knows health, wellness, balance, and good nutrition, and it is telling you what it needs at all times. Your job is to learn to trust it and follow its instructions.

What does relaxing on a tightrope mean? It means that we can rest on it, sleep on it, eat on it, watch TV on it, dance on it, shower on it, even have friends over and have a party on it. It means learning to have a full and well-rounded life every step of the way along our walk.

A useful mantra to achieve this state is:

Focus and flexibility.

Focus and freedom.

Focus and fun.

Let's now expand this image of a tightrope to include our entire path through life. From a larger perspective, your whole itinerary through existence could also be described as a wider tightrope. If we can learn to make ourselves relaxed, healthy, and balanced at this point of our tightrope walk, then we can also carry this ability into our daily lives, by creating the conditions where we feel at our best at every point of the journey.

Let's be clear: This does not mean that we won't meet disappointments, sadness, crises, heartbreak, and pain. There's no escaping the blues of life. We accept these as natural ingredients of what it means to be human. That said, within the parameters of life's organic cycles, we are not helpless. We can exercise control over our own well-being. Moreover, by regularly practicing healthy and life-affirming choices, we minimize bad things from occurring in our lives in the first place, and when they do occur—as bad things do happen to good people—we can deal with those crises in the best possible manner.

The System

Stretch your imaginary tightrope between where you are presently and where you want to be at the end. As mentioned earlier, this can be a physical destination, a mental state such as "I want to finish my master's degree," or a challenging situation you are currently facing that you would like to handle adroitly.

Clearly articulate to yourself the dangers lying on either side and below your tightrope.

Describe what scenario would constitute falling off this symbolic tightrope—what line you cannot cross.

Take stock of what property, belongings, instruments, and so on that you can have with you while you walk and live on this tightrope. See if you want to get rid of unnecessary stuff that has accumulated through the years without much thought. Remember: *The things you own, own you.* This is meant not as a prudish judgment of materialism but to encourage you to make this a conscious process. You do this not because "this is what everyone else does" but out of awareness that at every step of the way you have countless choices, and this is the decision you make for yourself.

Visualize yourself walking the rope comfortably and ask yourself what type of energy, approach, and conduct this tightrope walk will require in order to complete it successfully.

- What pace will you have to maintain?
- What can you afford to do, and what must you do without?
- Do you know how long this tightrope walk will last?
- What will you do if it has to last longer than you expect?
- Have you thought of alternatives in case of failure?

As with other exercises, the more answers you can have for possible different outcomes the better chances you will have to arrive at your desired destination.

Benefits

The primary benefit of this imagery sequence is that it teaches you to take superb care of yourself—right here and now. Because often you might not know how long you will need to stay on the tightrope, you'll have to develop the ability to be at your best at all times. This means listening to your body's needs, and providing it with sufficient rest, healthy nutrition, the ability to breathe freely at every moment, and an overall balanced lifestyle that satisfies the crucial components of your mind, body, and spirit.

This sequence makes you rid yourself of needless mental or physical baggage that might weigh you down. These may include:

- Thinking of material possessions as causes to happiness.
- Ascribing undue value to items that the outside world might consider important but to which your own instincts don't respond.
- Erroneous self-perception of things you thought you could not be or could not do.

This is a perfect moment; no moment will ever be more perfect than this.

If I can't learn to be happy in this moment, I'll never know happiness in my life.

Your Essence

Overview

Your life has a beginning point, an end point, and many connecting points in between. In this mental sequence, you stretch an imaginary through-line that links all these dots along your life span, and you notice the type of energy and approach that have gotten you from one point to another. This is your essence.

Applications

This mental structure combines spiritual, physical, philosophical, and emotional components to help you gain a clear image of yourself and the quality of energy that flowed through you during your passage through life.

When you see a clear through-line stretching between the different stations of your life, you know that you are living an authentic existence, traveling the path that you were meant to take. If, on the other hand, the path that you observe meanders and stalls in some sections, this could be a sign that significant life decisions on your part might be in order.

The System

You will begin by evoking the earliest recollection you have as a child. Then, you will recall a signature memory that you have from every decade of your life. You will end by visualizing yourself at the end point of your life. You will connect these various dots over your lifetime and observe this path from above to understand the spirit that drove you on your entire voyage.

Make yourself comfortable, and concentrate on your breath. Make sure that it is steady, even, and free.

Recall the earliest memory you have of yourself. The more details you are able to recollect, the more effective this exercise will be:

- How old are you?
- Where is this happening?
- Are you at home, or at someone else's place?
- Who is around you?
- How old are they?
- What time of the year is it?
- What is happening in this event you're recalling?

Remember how you feel at this occasion: Are you happy, distraught, or hungry?

Register in your mind the color and character of this experience.

Now recall the clearest occasion you have from your teens and follow the same questions that you used to refresh your childhood memory to see this remembrance in the most vivid detail.

Recollect the brightest memory you have from your twenties, and answer each of the questions above to help you create a strong and clear picture. Do the same to bring up a memory from your thirties. Follow this process until you arrive at the present moment—the person you are today.

Pause here for a second to take in the path you have traveled to get here: your past and present. You are that, but you're not *just* that. The remainder of your days are ahead of you. Your life does not stop today. Your complete identity also includes the yet-unrealized potential.

Now, sling your vision forward to the last day of your life and from there retrace your steps. Don't hesitate. State exactly how you want to depart life (for example, surrounded with your loved ones, having accomplished such and such, or at this or that location).

See what you are most proud of among the things you leave behind. Be as specific as you can. These details differ from person to person and all are valid, provided they are life-affirming.

Now, let your spirit exit your body. Hover over your body as in "out-of-body experience." Connect all the dots you've recalled along your life span, and see yourself walking the path you have outlined in your mind between past, present, and future.

- Who is the person walking?
- Who made the daily choices of what to wear, what to eat, where to go, and how to get there? Whom to meet, when to wake up, and when to go to bed?
- Who made the decision of the marriage proposal, the college you chose to attend, and the profession you are practicing?
- Who made those innumerable small and big decisions that have brought you to the present moment?
- What is the energy, the dominant feeling that you have from one point to the next?

That is your essence, the guiding spirit that is navigating your entire life.

Even if there were many diversions on this path, and drastic changes of direction, you take a view that is wide enough to include your entire life so you can see your overall through-line.

You contain many multitudes, but the overriding path through all those different points is your essence.

A related image that fits with this vision is the Arabic notion of *makhtub*: "It is written." In this view, everything in existence is predetermined. When we look back on our life, everything falls into place, everything makes sense. The wisdom of living a life forward well also consists in periodically stepping back and registering our entire journey as it unfolds in time and space.

Benefits

- Allows you a larger perspective of your being as it lifts your spirit from the mundane daily existence to envision your entire passage through life.
- Deepens your understanding of self and opens your imagination to include everything that you can be and do.
- Enables you to choose the type of journey you want to have through life as it shows you that the freedom and the responsibility to decide on the character of this voyage resides in you.

Your life is the canvas you are painting every day. It is good to step back occasionally to take in the entire picture.

Reverse Engineering/Future Pull

Overview

In this mental framework you visualize a future event that you want to see in your life, and you let that future pull you toward it. This event can be anything you desire (for example, winning an award, getting a better position at work, breaking an athletic record, learning to play the piano, writing a book, meeting the person of your dreams, or buying a beautiful house).

Applications

The easiest way to bring this vision about is to place yourself at your desired destination, look back, and retrace the important steps that have gotten you to this position. As you approach this sequence, consider the notion that in nature there are no punishments or rewards, only consequences. Every action creates a chain reaction and generates a fitting result.

As Chapter 4 noted, life in its essence is pure energy and intelligence. Everything in the universe vibrates as units of information, waves of probabilities floating in the ether of existence. Once we direct our attention, intention, and the effect of our actions on a particular probability, it has the potential to be set into place in the three-dimensional reality.

The System

Let's say for the purpose of this exercise that you want to become the branch manager of the bank in which you currently work as a junior executive.

Make yourself comfortable, grow quiet and centered, and establish a steady, even, effortless pattern of breaths.

Now see yourself clearly in the branch manager's position: You are sitting in the comfortable leather chair in the office; you are taking calls and checking the financial markets; you are helping others accomplish their tasks; you are solving problems; you are an asset to the bank; you like your new job; you are successful and happy.

Notice the color of the walls in the office; whether there are any paintings on the walls; the look and feel of the carpet or the floor.

In your mind, touch your desk and notice the important items you have on your desk when you are the branch manager. Be as specific as you can:

- What pictures, if any, are on your desk?
- Do you have a favorite pen?
- Do you use a laptop, a tablet, or a desktop computer?
- Approximately, how many people work at your branch?
- Do you have weekly meetings?
- Who do you report to, and who reports to you?

You are here, at your desired destination, established, solid, successful, and secure. Look back. How did you get here? Mentally retrieve the essential steps that have led you to this point in reality.

Register where you began: what your plan of action and your approach were, how you behaved with your coworkers, what you had to learn to personally advance to be qualified for this promotion, how you had to grow and develop as a competent manager.

Benefits

- Gives you an inventory of the inner resources of strength, competence, and imagination that you carry inside you.
- Teaches you invaluable discipline of detailed planning and precise execution.
- Shows you that the person ultimately responsible for your accomplishments in life is yourself.
- Helps you realize that as you'd imagined yourself at your desired position and created the conditions to get you there, in the same manner you can also create the conditions where you can be in the best physical and mental states at every day of your life.

Eye of the Storm

Overview

This sequence uses the mental image of a raging storm whose center is tranquil and still. No matter how loud and dangerous the circumstances outside of you, the eye of the storm within you is peaceful, steady, and safe.

Applications

This mental concept is best used in turbulent circumstances of any kind (work, family, bodily danger, a sport competition) in which it is vital for you to maintain a sense of composure and cool to resolve this crisis in a positive manner.

The System

You are dealing with an unpleasant event over which you have very little or no control. You are facing forces much larger than yourself. Your primary objective in this situation is to come out of it without physical or mental harm.

Drop in, and ride your breath into your center. Shift your mental focus from the storm raging around you to the peaceful place at your core.

This center of the storm that you're currently occupying—your inner world—is the most grounded place there is. It is anchored and planted in reality. You can feel it under your feet as a solid foundation that provides you with a stable support.

Now make a conscious choice to focus on your breath. This will be your mental switch to shift your attention from the negative event, over which you have no control, to a positive action, which you can monitor and regulate. This is your way to begin regaining your authority and strength in this situation: through your breath.

Here's a helpful phrase to use: *The only thing I can control is my own behavior, but that's plenty.*

See a mental image of yourself as a serene and levelheaded person passing through this storm of life and emerging on the other side in a healthy manner.

Follow your even and free breaths to guide you to the safe conclusion of this episode.

Benefits

- Helps you to locate a sense of discipline in yourself.
- Gives you a clear vision of your passage through life, in terms of what's under your influence and what's beyond your control.
- Gives you confidence that you can weather big storms of life in a self-respecting manner. The fact that you stayed

centered and calm during the storm means that you were able to tap your inner strength.

- Is a superb training for future crises and a tool for developing a sense of mastery at every point in your life.

Chess Game

Overview

This mental imagery technique uses the analogy of a chess game to help you make decisions in your life with the precision, wit, and shrewdness of a master tactician.

Applications

Think of yourself as an expert strategist who sees and plans their moves several steps ahead. You don't want to make your intentions obvious to others because you want to maintain the element of surprise. You want to be the one who is in the driver's seat, initiating events rather than responding to them. You will use your tactical skills of foresight, judgment, and careful planning to put into place a sequence of actions that will culminate in your desired outcome.

The System

This mental imagery is best used to deal efficiently with challenging situations in which strategic insight is essential. For example, you want to quit your job and you want to do this in the most favorable conditions for you:

- You don't want to burn any bridges behind you.
- You want to leave with a good severance package.
- You want to secure good references.
- And you want to ensure a smooth transition to your next position.

Like a master strategist in a chess game, you want to think through several moves ahead of every option available to you.

Benefits

- Teaches you to be cool, composed, and methodical in making decisions about important events in your life.
- Sharpens your skills of logical analysis, patience, and discipline.
- Increases your awareness and mastery of your available resources, whether they are chess pieces on the board or the finite amount of energy contained in your body.
- Improves your financial prudence, your ability to plan for the future, and your recognition of your powers. If you can systematically assess every situation to make the best-informed decision present at this time, then you can also create the conditions that enable you to be at your best at every stage of your life.

Navigating the 3D Grid of Life

Overview

The purpose of this mental picture is to enhance your consciousness of the three-dimensional nature of existence.

Applications

This imagery technique serves as a reminder that our passage through life consists of navigating a path in which various considerations, interests, factors, challenges, opportunities, and dangers lie below, above, to the left, to the right, and in every other direction around us in our proverbial flight through the open space of existence.

It is helpful here also to use the analogy of flight corridors for air traffic. Different planes are assigned different altitude and latitude routes for their flight, so at any given time there might be other airplanes that fly above, below, at a forty-five-degree angle to the left and above you, or a sixty-degree angle to the right and below you.

These metaphorical additional airplanes in your life can be other people's interests; game regulations of the sport you practice; code ethics of your profession (law procedures, medical protocol, or adhering to scientific research guidelines); your dependents' needs; traffic rules that you must obey; and so on. These are all parameters that you cannot violate for a safe passage through life for yourself and the people around you. Besides other persons' welfare, we also need to respect the fundamental laws of nature for a secure and graceful journey through the matrix of life.

The System

Imagine yourself flying in midair, surrounded on all sides by entities and objects at the full spectrum of 360 degrees: above, below, left, right, and various degrees of angles in between.

For example: You are sitting in your car in morning traffic at 7 a.m. heading for work.

- Above you there's the rude cashier at the store who gave you your cup of coffee thirty minutes earlier.
- Below you is the mortgage payment, which concerns you and which is due at the end of the month.
- Ahead of you is the traffic accident that you know will make you late for work.
- Behind you is last night's argument with your spouse that is still nagging at you since it was not resolved in a satisfactory manner.
- To the left of you is the declining health of your mother.
- And to the right of you is your own toothache, which you hope will not develop into a full-blown emergency.

What is the most life-affirming path through this situation?

Align the energies inside you with those outside, so you can pass through life with the least amount of friction.

What does this mean in practical terms? It means listening to your body and heart to understand exactly what you feel, and what causes you to feel this way, and then finding a resolution that will put you in a position where you will feel most comfortable mentally, physically, and emotionally. This can be a challenging and time-consuming mission, but this is also a part of being alive.

As I said earlier, we determine the quality and quantity of our life span by the small choices we make every day. Our enjoyable and fulfilling path through existence is something that no one can give to us but us. This is a license and a responsibility that reside inside us—a gift we give to ourselves.

Benefits

- Sharpens your perception of the marvelous complexity of life and improves your ability to operate with precision and skill.
- Gives you a better understanding of your individual position in the larger framework of existence.
- Improves your awareness of the interconnectedness and interdependence of the world inside you and the world outside.

Not every mental imagery technique covered here will be right for you, nor will it be right for every challenge you encounter. However, the more instruments you carry in your mental toolkit, the more solutions you'll have to life's different problems.

The latest neuroscience shows that the conscious mind is in charge of our activities roughly 5 percent of the time. The subconscious mind is responsible for 95 percent of our life's experiences. The way the subconscious operates is that in the future a certain event that you'll face will trigger a memory of one of the thirteen mental imagery tools that you acquired here, and will bring it to the forefront of your psyche. At that point, you'll be able to recall the particular system of this mental imagery tool and it will help you to handle the situation that you're facing in a satisfactory manner.

Listen to the flow of life inside you; listen to the force of life inside you; listen to the rhythm of your body; listen to the rhythm of the world.

CHAPTER TWELVE

Sensing Your Duration

By now, we have established in the book that the potential to sense the amount of energy our body contains clearly exists in the consciousness of the universe and in our own genetic makeup. We have examined the scientific foundations of this perception. We have looked back to the origins of life as we currently understand them, and we looked forward to possible future developments of humankind on this planet. We have gazed out into the edge of the cosmos to see the relationships of galaxies, planets, and stars. And we brought that large cosmos back into our own body to see that this celestial body of flesh, blood, and bones is in its essence made of the same energy and intelligence, and is governed by the same natural laws, which regulate all life in the universe.

As has been noted in Chapter 10, the latest medical studies describe the relationship that genes and lifestyle choices play in determining a person's longevity as roughly 30 to 70 percent in favor of lifestyle choices.[1] Our family history is an important element in determining our approximate life span, but the crucial factor that influences the quality and quantity of our life is our behavior. Your father might have lived one hundred years, and your mother might have lived 105 years. If you have no major ailments you have the potential to live about the same amount of years.

However, if you smoke, eat unhealthy, or abuse your body in other ways, you naturally shorten that potential significantly.

Let's also refresh the difference between longevity and life span. Longevity refers to the ongoing efforts to extend the amount of years humans live. Human longevity has been increasing at a rate of about two years per decade. Longevity implies a lengthy life. Lifespan, on the other hand, refers to a given amount of years a person lives—whether it is short or long. Life span is a neutral term, describing an overall duration of a person's life.

The highest knowledge I can gain in this existence is self-awareness. When I understand myself I understand the world.

In his monumental work (of 786 pages) from 1992, *The Future of the Body*, Michael Murphy, co-founder of Esalen Institute, which was an early bridgehead in the 1960s for Eastern wisdom traditions in the United States and a pioneer in the human potential movement, writes:

> When we have a spiritual insight that lifts us to certitudes we have not experienced before, or when we surprise ourselves by accomplishing some extraordinary deed, we might say that "something came over us," that we were "carried away." The recognition of ego-transcendent powers is reflected in religious terms and in our common language. That recognition of a Something beyond, I propose, coupled with our inability to specify its operations in us, points toward a new kind of human development. We don't know where our new vision, love, or joy came from, or how we effected our marvelous deed, precisely because such things are unfamiliar and because their mediations are related to something emergent in us.[2]

That was twenty-six years ago, and you and I are able to talk now about our latent capacity to sense how long we can live thanks to the insights and discoveries found in that and other books that came before this one. This is another clear sign of evolution—of our minds, of science, of the universe.

How do we know anything exists? By experiencing it through our senses. We see, hear, feel, touch, taste, and through these experiences we come to know an object.

How do we sense? What is the mechanism by which we touch, let's say, a velvet cloth with our hands and by which that action translates into a perception and feeling of softness and lushness in our mind and body? Our sense receptors (eyes, ears, mouth, fingers) are the portals through which experience enters our brain, which serves as the processing center. In *The Brain that Changes Itself*, Norman Doidge writes, "All our sense receptors translate different kinds of energy from the external world, no matter about the source, into electrical patterns that are sent down our nerves. These electrical patterns are the universal language "spoken" inside the brain—there are no visual images, sounds, smells, or feelings moving inside our neurons."[3]

We currently are aware of five senses: smell, vision, touch, hearing, and taste. Doidge writes, "We have senses we don't know we have—until we lose them; balance is one that normally works so well, so seamlessly, that it is not listed among the five that Aristotle described and was overlooked for centuries afterward."[4] In addition to the basic senses of sight, hearing, touch, taste, and smell we also have more recently revealed senses of temperature, balance, and vibration.[5]

As has been pointed out previously, we have not completed our evolution as a species. As long as life continues, and as long as the universe exists, we will keep discovering new capacities in ourselves and out in the cosmos. From previously seeing the brain as fixed and hardwired by the end of childhood, neuroscience has come to view the brain as a malleable, multipurpose organ that adjusts itself to the environment and our developing personal needs. Because we humans are much weaker physically than many animal species living on the planet, we wouldn't have survived and wouldn't have come to dominate our environment if our brains had not been adaptable and plastic. As Doidge writes, "(nature) has given us a brain that survives in a changing world by changing itself."[6]

As also noted previously, your body stores memories of everything you have experienced, good and bad. When you need to make a decision, a network of myriad sensory triggers in your body recalls what it would be like to decide this way or that. All this happens involuntarily, subconsciously, in fragments of seconds. All your past experiences carry physical markers in your body. When decision time comes, these memories instantaneously come to the surface. This is your mental library of intellectual, physical, and sensory impressions that steer you through life.

Before you begin the exercise of sensing your optimal duration, you need to do two things:

1. Have a full physical evaluation (heart rate, blood pressure, any existing conditions you might have).
2. Research your family history (longevity, proclivity toward certain illnesses, medical conditions that run in the family, and any other information that will help you understand your genetic makeup).

These two requirements will increase your knowledge of your mind-body-energy, and will help you to identify in yourself the amount of years you could reasonably last in this lifetime. The emphasis for you is that this number is sensible and logical, that it fits within the parameters of your family history, and at the same time agrees with your own condition.

In the following exercise you access your heart, mind, and intuition, as you draw inside to your core and touch the center of your being. You want to use the simplest and most direct way that gets you attuned with your body, and that is through your breath.

Being attuned to your body means listening to its metabolism and rhythm, identifying whether it's tired, hungry, thirsty, or sluggish. As we have seen, these are all signals that the body communicates to us regularly and continuously. You want to begin this exercise when your body is in its optimal condition (that is, when the communication channels to your center are clear). It's good to mention that the word *intuition* comes from the Latin *intuir,* meaning "knowledge from within."

Exercise: Sensing Your Body's Rhythm and Duration

Get comfortable in your chair, and establish a free and steady pattern of breaths. Inhale, exhale—nice, effortless breaths.

See if you want to stretch, yawn, or roll your shoulders to loosen.

The goal of this exercise is to help you recognize your inner tempo, and the best way to do this is by listening to your heartbeat.

Drop in and do a mental checklist of each part of your body.

Begin with the parts farthest away from your head. Notice how the toes on your left foot feel.

Then the right foot.

Now your ankles. Do they feel tight or loose?

Your calves, left and right.

Your shins.

Your knees.

Take your time; don't rush.

Let's move up to your pelvis, then abdomen.

Pay attention to how your chest feels.

See if you want to roll your shoulders, or lift them up and drop them down to release any lingering tension.

Now let's go up to your head, and tap gently on the top of your head. This is your crown.

Now down to your forehead. You can massage each part gently as we name them here.

And your eyebrows.

Let's go down to your ears.

Now lightly touch your cheeks.

Your jaw.

Your chin.

Drop your mouth down like in a comfortable yawn and move your jaw around softly to release any tension you might have there.

Now go down to your neck.

And back to your shoulders.

Now go down to your chest, where you previously placed that glowing sun at the center of your heart.

Pay attention to your breath. Make sure that it is steady and free.

Grow quiet in this place and listen to your heart beat.

Now consider the fact that every kind of animal has a unique frequency and quality of energy, and identifying these helps us understand our own natural tempo.

Ask yourself:

- If I were an animal, what animal would I be?
- Do I have the rhythm of a giraffe, or a cat, or a bird, or a dog?
- If I were a dog, what breed would I be? A golden retriever, a Rottweiler, maybe a greyhound, or a Jack Russell?
- If I were a bird, what kind would I be? A crow, or a pelican, a hummingbird, or maybe an owl?
- Am I maybe a tiger, or a horse, a deer, or a wolf?
- Which of these animals operates at the frequency that is most similar to mine?

Continue to breathe steady and free, and also consider that your breath and your heartbeat are interconnected and interdependent just like your body and mind are inseparable parts of you.

You are starting to identify your internal rhythm, and from here we'll gradually move toward locating in yourself your optimal duration of existence.

Now choose from the techniques that we covered in this book the one that's your favorite. It can be a pressure point exercise, a meditation routine, a mental imagery tool, a touch trigger, or a combination of several of those. Here and elsewhere, keep this process simple: The first technique that comes to mind is normally the one that has resonated with you the most.

I'll be guiding you every step of the way, and you and I will keep our feet firmly on the ground to lead you to where you can start to identify your optimal duration in yourself. At the end of this process, there's no outside governing authority that hands out a signed certificate that says, "We hereby declare that you shall live 104 years and ninety-five days." Rather, this governing authority resides in you. You will recognize in yourself a number according to your awareness of your physical and mental states—and this figure will make sense as the duration that you can reasonably live in your body. This number is a potential that you will be able to realize by the choices you make in your daily life.

To clarify this point with a personal example: I'm operating from the premise that if I behave in a certain way and treat my body and mind in a certain way, I can last in this lifetime for 102 years. This doesn't mean that accidents can't happen. I know that they can. I also recognize that in the universe there are forces much larger than myself, and this gives me a sense of humility to not grow arrogant. But within the framework over which I have control—my own behavior—I know that I can sustain life in this body for 102 years. At that time I'll have completed my life's journey.

This understanding of the energy in my body gives me a sense of confidence, clarity, and stability, and it makes me realize that I am in charge of my passage through life with the choices I make every day. As we said, understanding our optimal duration is only the first part of the equation. The other crucial part is applying the self-management skills that would make that potential come true.

Mind-body medicine pioneer Larry Dossey writes in his 2007 book *The Extraordinary Healing Power of Ordinary Things*, "Several studies show that what one *thinks* about one's health is one of the most accurate predictors of longevity ever discovered (emphasis in original)."[7] Common sense also says that longer is not necessarily better. Don't aim for a higher rather than a lower number to emerge. It is the quality and not the quantity of life that counts. Follow this mantra: Don't push. Allow.

Now make sure that your breath is even and free and consider these points:

Faith is an essential component in locating my optimal duration, but this faith is based on clear understanding of myself and of how the world operates.

Do I know that this will happen? No. The nature of "knowing" is that we can't know what hasn't happened yet. But if it were to happen, this is how it would: through what I think and how I act.

As mentioned earlier, the longest verified human life on record is 122 years. Even without accounting for the anticipated increase in human life span, within these known boundaries, any reasonable number that I can conceive according to my physical and mental states is valid.

Would I want to live forever? No, that would be tedious and pointless. Life is precious because it is finite.

If I can recognize how long I can live, how would that account for illnesses and diseases? The correct way to think about this is that this is not a guarantee, but a *potential* that might come true if I make certain decisions.

It will only happen if I can create the conditions in which I can be the best version of myself at every age.

Let me ask myself a practical question:

- *If it were to happen,* how would I have to behave?
- How would I have to think?
- How would I have to breathe?
- Exercise?
- Eat? And what not to eat?
- How would I have to pace myself thru the distance that I'm seeing?

My power lies in accepting that the freedom and responsibility for my overall wellness are in my hands.

We strive for certainties, but are obliged to operate within the structure of educated risks and prudent hopes. All life consists of making the best choices out of less-than-perfect data. However, we know the basics:

It's better not to smoke, it's better not to be overweight, it's better not to have addictions, it's better to stay physically and mentally active.

So, out of the big void of uncertainty, I carve for myself a framework of consciousness, that says: *This is how long I can exist in this world, and I support this decision with everyday choices.*

Make sure that you're breathing steady and free, and also consider this: Granted, I don't know many things about the universe, but let this fact not paralyze me from acting on what I do know: understanding my body's needs and creating the best conditions for it.

My body knows health, longevity, and balance, and communicates these to me on a regular basis.

I'm made of the same ingredients that make up the stars and the planets. By trusting my body's intuition, I trust universal intelligence.

I come from the source of life, and I return to the source of life when I complete my physical journey.

Growing up and growing old is not a drawback but a natural cycle like the changing seasons. I can't prevent one or the other, but what I *can* do is make sure that I'm the best version of myself at every age.

Pay attention to your breath, make sure there's no tension in your body, and also consider this: The spirit in you is ageless. It enters your body for a duration when you're born, drives you through your life span, and then rejoins its source.

What will you be after you die? What you were before you were born. If you can conceive of that past, you can also imagine that future.

Can you address the eternal in you? The essence that will remain after your body is gone? Can you own up to that identity? Here is a mantra to help you get there: I live here, I live everywhere, now and forever.

You are as much a drop in the cosmic ocean of existence as this entire ocean is contained in you.

The genetic information in your body carries memories of every life-form you've been along your evolutionary path.

The currents flowing through your body are not only energy and matter but also time and space.

Like the universe itself, you're constantly changing and evolving. Ask yourself:

- Where do I see myself five years from now?
- Ten years?
- Twenty years?
- Can I imagine myself at eighty? Ninety? A hundred?
- Do I *want* to live to eighty? Ninety? A hundred?
- What would it take for me to live to eighty? Ninety? A hundred?
- What would I have to do?
- What would I have to avoid doing?
- How would I have to treat myself?
- How would I have to treat others?
- How would I have to monitor my health over that entire distance?
- Are there any changes that I'd have to make from my current lifestyle, or do I like where my path is leading? (Remember: This is your life, and nobody can dictate what you do with it.)

Reflect on your plans, dreams, and ambitions in the world.

Keep breathing steady and free, and consider this, too:

Sensing how long I can live also means that the consciousness that is *I*, my personal identity, can master my mind, body, and spirit for the duration that I'm seeing.

A finite amount of gas has been poured into the tank of my existence. How will I divide this energy over the entire distance of my journey? Like in a car, if I drive very fast, accelerate rapidly, and break suddenly, I burn more gas.

Without passing judgment one way or the other—as long as you don't harm yourself or others—the more you understand your vehicle the better you'll be able to control it.

When you know the amount of energy you have, then you can manage this life force like a faucet that you turn on and off to regulate the flow of water.

At home, after you'd done your medical exam and your family's lifespan research, you'll end all these questions with the following one: Considering what I've learned from my checkup and from the longevity history of my family, how long do I think I can reasonably live in this body?

Don't rush or anticipate any outcome. Simply listen to the reactions that this question generates in your body. When you begin to sense your optimal duration, see how this figure fits in the overall framework of your life.

It's good here to attach a touch trigger to this number to help you in future meditations.

Recall the Future Pull mental imagery tool. You've reached the age you've sensed for yourself. Now look back. How did you get here? What choices did you make to get to this age? What was the energy and approach driving you through life?

You can also see your current position in the perspective of your larger journey, and this will give you a sense of stability by realizing that your present station in life is an organic part of your whole existence.

Ask yourself: *Now that I have a sense of how long I can live, does that scare me because it makes death more real, or does it empower and enlighten me, because now I'm in full control of my time on Earth?*

Sensing your optimal duration also means that every cell and fiber in your body, and also everything you think and do, agrees with the duration you've seen for yourself. This is a mental, physical, emotional, and spiritual framework: the structure of your life.

If no number appears for several sessions, don't worry and don't feel disappointed. This means that you're not yet at the stage in which this awareness can naturally come to the surface. Simply continue with your favorite exercises and continue developing your intuition. Remember: This is not a quick fix but a road map. You're on a journey of self-discovery, and, like a good explorer, you need to be patient, be prudent, and enjoy the ride.

Repeat this exercise periodically, whether you're in bed, walking, or exercising, until the awareness of your optimal duration slowly emerges in you. Remember the mantra: Don't push. Allow. Not only can you do it, but this is how it's done: by listening to your body and trusting what it tells you.

Your body contains the entire information of existence, and will give you all the answers when you listen. Your body knows.

CHAPTER THIRTEEN

Framework of Your Life

Now that we've identified in ourselves our optimal duration of existence, let's set in place a master structure for our life that will enable us to harness the energies of our body and mind and use them in the best possible manner.

Let's also set in place a few guideposts: Life is sacred. Good life means different things to different people. However, basic ingredients need to be present in every enjoyable life: health, meaning, the feeling that one is loved and valued, adequate conditions of living, and for most people, having a significant other.

This chapter will guide you in establishing your own framework of life, which will give you a sense of stability, clarity, confidence, meaning, ease, and balance—according to your individual personality, ambitions, needs, and overall approach to life.

Picture this mental image: Just like a new building being erected, your structure of life consists of its eventually invisible foundations below ground and four visible panels above ground: left, right, front, and back. Each of these four planks is a conceptual guidepost you set for your journey through existence. They can be your dreams, goals, relationships, principles, or anything else you consider vital and dear for a satisfying passage through life.

Just like erecting a skyscraper, the taller you want to go up, the deeper you'll have to go down. In other words, if you set yourself high goals, they will have to be supported by solid foundations inside you. Build your base of your most durable materials—your best qualities of faith, passion, courage, intelligence, patience, goodness, commitment, and any special talent you have—so they can be your steady support and help you withstand life's toughest challenges.

For the purpose of erecting your master structure of life, going deep into the ground to plant dependable foundations also means asking yourself the honest questions of what is really important in your life, and why. When you understand the reasons of why you do what you do, these answers will be the stable bedrock on which you'll be able to build the tall and beautiful building of your life.

Once this master structure is standing, its planks will be the leading parameters of your life. Not only will they not restrict or hem you in, but on the contrary: They'll serve as the guideposts to where your energy can flow with purpose and ease. These are the clear lines where your attention, time, effort, and passion can be channeled in the desired direction.

As every adult person learns, life can be complex and filled with multiple simultaneous interrelated considerations. The five planks that you select for your master structure are not your attempt to trivialize or reduce life's complexities, but a way to establish the essential components on which all the other important factors of your life will rest. In times of crises, or when you need to make big decisions in your life, these five vital elements will help you to quickly re-orient yourself toward your true path through life.

This intelligent structure will also prevent you from desperate and reckless actions, as it will outline the boundaries of a healthy and enjoyable life. You will establish flexible, comfortable, and livable panels in which you will have plenty of room to move around and breathe freely, and that will protect you during your entire journey through existence.

To help you get a clear idea of this sequence, here is a description of my master structure of life: Whatever I do, I will always make life-affirming choices; I'll be a loving husband, a considerate brother, a good example for my students, workshop participants, and readers by the way I live my life; and I will aim to give full expression to the skills and talents I've been given by my creator. To me, this constitutes a happy and fulfilling life.

We begin with the bottom panel: the *foundation* of existence, which supports the entire scaffolding of life. This could be your overriding philosophy—your creed. In my case it looks like this:

Bottom panel: Life-affirming choices

Whatever I think and do will serve rather than harm life. In every-day situations this commitment also guides me to breathe and be present through frustrations, annoyances, and other unpleasant circumstances. To not do anything rash that would be regrettable later on, but simply to breathe and pass through this moment as I regain my inner peace and clarity. My solid rock of existence is that life is sacred, I have been granted a portion of this life for a duration, and I am determined to make the most of this precious gift.

Left panel: Loving husband

Whatever actions I take in life and whatever I refrain from doing, I will remain a good and thoughtful husband to my wife.

Right panel: Considerate brother

I will behave in such a way that my sister can always know how much I love and appreciate the person that she is.

Front panel: Good example for my students, workshop participants, and readers

Here I am guided by the age-old maxim that the best and only way to teach others is by personal example.

Back panel: Full expression to the skills and talents I've been given

I believe that each of us comes into life with a unique gift, and the secret to a fulfilled existence lies in realizing this potential both for our own reward and to make the largest contribution in the world.

Foundations, left, right, front, and back are the panels that every typical building contains, capped by the top panel, the roof. However, in your master structure of life this top panel is left open. To signify your continuous growth, unlimited potential, and the pragmatic acknowledgment that from today's perspective you can't possibly see what the future holds, you allow for exciting and positive developments in your life and in life in general. Your past and present are not your entire narrative; your whole future is ahead of you.

Exercise: Establishing Your Master Structure

Let's now begin to establish your master scaffolding of life. It is best to do this exercise with a pen and paper, a smartphone, or a tablet, so you can make notes to yourself as you go.

Lie or sit down in your favorite position at a comfortable place at home or outside where you won't be disturbed.

Grow quiet and concentrate on your breath.

Make sure that your breath is free, effortless, steady, and deep.

Center yourself by drawing into your core, and slowly start making a personal checklist. Ask yourself:

- What are the essential components of my life?
- What is non-negotiable?
- What needs to be present in my existence without which I cannot do? Be patient and genuine with answering this question because this is the essence of your structure. Every time you come up with an answer that strikes a chord in you, write it down.
- Over the entire life span I can see for myself, what must I have? Wealth? Fame? Love? Satisfaction? Thrills? Meaning?
- If it's wealth, what level of prosperity do I need to have to feel safe and satisfied?
- If it's satisfaction, what type of fulfillment am I looking for?
- Do I want appreciation? Self-esteem?
- What are my ambitions?

- What am I willing to do to realize these ambitions?
- Do I need to live out all my dreams, desires, urges?
- Do I want peace of mind, and what will give me this peace of mind where I can be content with what I am right now?
- Do I have the love that I want in my life?
- If not, is there anything that I need to do in terms of personal development to create the situation where I can attract my ideal partner?
- What are my most sacred goals, without which I won't feel that I'd lived a happy life?
- What do I want my existence to stand for?
- Is it important for me to leave some kind of legacy?
- Is it important for me to leave property to my loved ones?

Reflect on these questions, and make sure you are relaxed and breathing deeply and freely.

As with every other exercise in this book, the more specific questions you ask yourself and the more authentic answers you'll find for them, the more tangible benefits they will give you in your everyday existence. This is because the process of understanding what really resonates with you helps to focus your energies, attention, skills, talents, and efforts onto the truly important things in your life, and helps set you on the path of accomplishing them.

Now, from all the good answers that you've written about the important things in your life, whittle this list down to five crucial items—items without which you cannot do. This will be your master structure in life.

Next, select from among the five key points on your list the one that is absolutely vital to your being. This is your bottom panel: the single most important principle that supports all the others—your foundation in life—and follow it with left panel, then right, front, and back.

Leave the top panel open as a symbol of your growth and infinite potential. You understand that your life goes on and you evolve with it, and if and when the time comes, you'll replace a plank that you had erected in your master scaffolding with a new one that will make more sense in your life in the future. This is part of the fluid and open nature of existence and of your own limitless potential.

When you set these panels in place—when you articulate to yourself the vital planks of your framework of life—make the headlines plain and memorable. First form a short-hand version of the panel, a brief phrase that conveys the pure idea of your principle, and then elaborate on it in a few sentences.

The distilled version of your individual guidepost will also serve as a perfect touch trigger to plant in your body so later you can easily recall it at will. You can plant all five planks at different locations, and this mind-body process will help you deepen the new consciousness of your optimal duration of existence and the sound master structure you have erected for yourself. Keep this process practical and simple. You want to be able to use it in your daily life without much effort.

As you build this solid foundation, be sure to include among the building blocks in your framework of life a sense of gentleness toward yourself, so if you periodically fall short of the personal standards you had set for your behavior, you can forgive yourself and make this a learning experience. A growing mastery of your inherent resources implies that you are not overly harsh on yourself and understand that you, like the universe, are a work in progress. As long as you aim to be the best version of yourself at every stage of the journey you are headed in the right direction.

It is also important to maintain flexibility in your master structure. As in a skyscraper, it should withstand strong winds and hurricanes and, rather than crack or buckle, it should gently sway with the oncoming elements of nature. The wisdom of graceful passage through existence also consists in adapting to the unpredictable conditions of life while staying true to our inner character.

The most evident benefit that your master scaffolding provides for dealing with stressful events that regularly crop up in life is a sense of balance and perspective. When you face a daunting situation, you may tell yourself, "This is a difficult time. I am in a tight spot. I feel overwhelmed by the enormity of the challenges facing me. However, as I know from my larger framework of life, I have another X amount of years ahead of me, so I will put this incident in the proper context and pace myself through the entire journey of my life."

Structure of life = mastery and meaning.

Managing Time

Sometimes people say that they "don't have enough time," that they "don't know where time went," or that their "time just slips through the fingers." In these cases, it is helpful to realize that just as the body contains a finite amount of energy, so the agreed-upon construct of a twenty-four-hour-a-day cycle also consists of a given amount of time. To sharpen this point, when a person feels that they cannot manage time, this is an indication that they are not able to properly manage their inner resources of energy, attention, breath, and effort.

Life is precious because it is finite. Having a sound master structure in our life enables us to gain control of our time, because now we clearly see our potential duration of existence and can choose how to distribute our energy, breath, and effort over the full span of our lifetime. In essence, mastery of our time equals mastery of our self.

Managing Money

Money is a form of congealed energy. Its common representation is in paper or metal currency, bank and government notes, and other instruments accepted by society to ascribe value to things and to conduct commerce. On a personal level, its value and meaning lie in enabling us to translate into existence what our mind conjures and desires. Of course, money cannot realize everything that the mind wants. This is an inherent characteristic of money as being a form of static energy, and just as not every fanciful item that the mind wants can be brought into existence, so money is limited in its power to create every outcome.

Because money is a form of raw energy, managing money efficiently means managing our inner resources in a conscious and competent manner. When a person "runs out of money," "can't make ends meet," and "lives beyond their means," these unfortunate situations indicate their lack of self-management skills—of finances, energy, time, and efforts.

If you are currently in a situation in which you don't feel in full control of your finances, return to the master structure you have established in your life, and change one of the essential panels in your framework to a panel of fiscal responsibility. In this panel, you'll commit yourself to not let your financial situation to get out of hand. This is not an easy process, and will require of you honesty, discipline, maturity, and prudence. But in order for us to gain independence in life we have to be accountable for our actions, because this is the only way that we are able to rise to our full potential.

Tell yourself: Others have done this and I can do this as well. Make a deliberate choice to think of money as your friend and not an enemy, a stranger, or a mysterious entity that you cannot comprehend. Remember: Money is just another form of your energy. There's nothing to fear. It is a tool, an extension of your power. When we understand our powers, we simply take account of the money we have as one of several factors in the overall framework of our life. You have a finite amount of money in your bank, of time in your day, and of heartbeats and energy in your body. It is up to you to decide how to use them with the priorities you establish in your life. If you decide that having a large amount of money is absolutely essential to your life, you will also be able to accomplish this, as many others have done, by adjusting your intention, attention, and actions onto this particular purpose.

Overcoming Fears

There are two dominant feelings when we approach every decision: faith and fear in varying proportions, and the degree to which one overcomes the other largely determines the outcome of our actions.

Fear is an organic part of life, like breath, love, hate, curiosity, happiness, and hunger. In most cases, when people don't admit to being afraid they only show their fear of being frightened. In fact, this is the most pernicious aspect of fear, that it scares an individual into burying their fear deep inside themselves to the point in which it becomes a dark secret that they're reluctant to acknowledge. There is nothing weak or dishonorable about conceding that we are frightened; life with its many uncertainties can be a terrifying business. However, the key to a brave and meaningful existence lies in the way we deal with our natural fears.

It is important here to realize that just like hate, curiosity, or happiness, fear does not occur anywhere except in the mind, and like any other thought held in the mind, it can be managed, subdued, or changed. It does not exist per se in the world but is a construct of the subjective reality we are observing and can be amended when we alter how we look at our surroundings.

We conquer our fears by first acknowledging them, accepting them as a part of what makes us the particular individuals we are, embracing this part of ourselves, then looking the fear squarely in the face and understanding what gives it the power that it holds over us.

For a long-lasting solution we cannot go around this fear, brush it away, or bury it. It will eventually surface as an unresolved baggage. But in this very action of embracing this fear lies the resolution to the problem: Our fear will burn and melt away when we have the courage to address it honestly and fully. Ask yourself: *What is the worst outcome of this situation? What do I fear the most that will happen?* Following this question, you need to have the humble conviction that you will accept the consequences of whatever outcome will result. Your acceptance of the responsibility for your fears leads you to realize that you are much bigger than your fears. Your mind has created them, and your mind can also dissolve them. Tell yourself: I am responsible for my actions, and I am smart and strong enough to understand this fear, grow stronger from it, and go forward with my healthy life regardless of what this fear does.

As fear does not exist anywhere else but in the mind, so stress is a result of an individual's inner reaction. We have no control over what another person will do, or what circumstances we will face. We do have control over how we will react to every situation we experience.

The magical thing about addressing a frightful situation in an honest manner is that the fear that we conquer gives us its power. If we can find a satisfactory reply to the problem we faced that means we are now that much stronger for it.

What else do you think you cannot do while you are alive?

The energy and intelligence of the cosmos inform every cell in your body.

Making Tough Decisions

The older I grow the stronger I grow, because I understand myself better.

If you feel that your life at present is out of balance and that you need to make difficult and important decisions to steer your life in a better direction, here are a few thoughts that will assist you with this challenge.

It takes as much effort to live a brave life as a timid one so you may as well do something that you really want.

Once you've understood that there is a given amount of time that you will exist in this world, any actions that you take—whether they take you away from your goals or bring you closer to them—will fill the same span of time allotted to you on earth.

From this perspective, whatever you do uses the same quantity of your precious time and energy. Have the humble faith in yourself and your creator to follow your most sacred dream.

Ask yourself: *What do I truly want in life?* This is exactly what your maker wants for you. The satisfaction we experience in life is intrinsically linked to the courage that we are able to summon to pursue our deepest yearnings.

Proud humility and humble pride: humility to do the job, and pride in knowing you are second to none.

If you've been feeling depressed for a while, you must seek help from a medical professional to address the specific circumstances that led to this condition. If, however, you've been experiencing a period of general unease or dissatisfaction that you haven't been able to understand, sometimes it is helpful to think of these feelings as the psyche's way to prompt us to make adjustments in our lives.

These times of discontent are often indicators of imbalances in a person's life, such as unfulfilled ambitions, in which the psyche recognizes that the visible life that a person is living does not correspond to the internal aspirations of the heart and mind; being lonely; dealing with health problems; a feeling of being at a dead-end professionally, socially, or romantically; and a broad sense of unhappiness where one feels that the negatives in their life outweigh the positives.

To begin restoring equilibrium among the mental, physical, and spiritual aspects in one's life, it is useful to recall the image of an elevator: Going up means reaching the higher realms of our psyche; going down means reaching the bottom of our core. In this analogy, reaching the lowermost of one's psyche is a welcome position, because that is where the base of our being is located. This is the stable ground on which we can build our overall wellness. We need to arrive at our lowermost roots, because this is where we pour the foundations of our master structure in life.

In this sense, what is called "depression" can be more accurately described as "correction." As the psyche's natural correcting mechanism, this period of discomfort can be an education and preparation for the next stage in a person's development. It is an opportunity for honest self-assessment, realization of deep truths about oneself, and a strengthening of one's hold on existence. To revisit the image of a skyscraper that you erect as your structure, the higher you aim to build your life, the deeper you need to build its foundations.

No one can be a better you than you. Your gift of a lifetime is to understand what makes you the unique individual you are. This is your special place in the world. It will be to your benefit as well as the benefit of the cosmos if you can live your most authentic and fulfilled life.

CHAPTER FOURTEEN

Changing Bad Habits to Good Ones

Due to the marketplace forces of commercial interests, health insurance practices, technological advances in diagnostic equipment, and a general movement toward specialization, today's medical profession focuses mainly on the causes of physical disease rather than on the causes of physical health. The modern healthcare approach is largely symptom-focused and reactive rather than prevention-focused and proactive. Physicians seldom discuss with their patients basic components of a healthy and balanced life, such as nutrition, exercise, and lifestyle modification, and instead primarily address the diagnosis and treatment of disease. This stems from the fact that most clinicians are not trained to help patients incorporate relaxation, stress management, or mind-body practices into their daily lives, practices that naturally enhance the body's immune system.

This book's aim is not to discount the necessary role that medicine plays over the entire span of a person's life, but rather to amplify the primary role that each individual plays in their own wellness. Because our body is a combined product of our genetic makeup, our thought processes, and our behavior patterns, the person most responsible for our overall well-being is ourselves.

When we decide to replace in our lives bad habits with better ones, it's helpful to keep in mind a few basic principles:

- The greatest hurdle that most individuals face when they come to the nitty-gritty of changing their habits is to apply what their mind has understood to be correct and beneficial into specific choices in their everyday lives. This is the essence of the mind-body connection, and the crucial step that needs to happen to assimilate what we've learned into our daily routines.

- As a general rule, one can't simply eliminate a bad habit and leave a vacuum where it had been. This space needs to immediately be filled with a good healthy activity.

- If, as we saw in Chapter 5, the brain continues to change through our entire life span, this means that our approach to life and our behavior can also change. Our brain is not set in stone, nor is our personality, because we have the ability to learn from past mistakes and improve our approach to life as we go along.

- Our lives are based on our perceptions of the world and of ourselves. But our perceptions can be right or wrong. In that aspect, they're more accurately described as beliefs. We can change our beliefs by changing our way of thinking.

- Every minute approximately one million cells in your body die and are replaced by an equivalent number of new cells. Your old cells, containing negative beliefs and behaviors, leave your body and you can substitute them with new beliefs and behaviors that are more conducive to your health and well-being.

- "Letting go" rather than "getting rid" of bad habits: Realize both in body and in mind that *there are certain substances that you simply do not need to survive.* Your body requires food and water to exist, and it needs oxygen to breathe, but substances such as nicotine and other drugs are *simply not essential for your survival.*

- The fundamental factor in a person being able to change their habits is for them to change their perception of themselves—their beliefs about what they are capable of doing, and their overall awareness of their mind, body, and spirit.

- The human brain is naturally programmed to evolve, transform, and configure new connections between the billions of nerve cells it contains throughout our entire life span. This process is called neurogenesis: The brain produces new neurons until the day we die.

- This means that we can keep the mind active and sharp well into the higher decades of our life by keeping ourselves stimulated with mental, physical, and spiritual pursuits.

Recall that the superstring theory/unified field (see Chapter 4) show that at the essence of all existence are units of fluctuating information, vibrating strings of energy and intelligence, that collapse into reality according to the observer and the anticipated outcome that observer is projecting onto them. This inherent pliability of the universe tells us that there are no real facts in life, only perceptions. We don't see objects as they are; we see them as our experience has taught us to see them. We create our worlds by what we think about what we see; we explain to ourselves in our minds what we are observing, and through this figuring-out process we arrive at certain conclusions about the world around us and our place in it.

Our belief systems about the world and about ourselves form the boundaries of what we think we can and cannot do. This process begins in our mind, and this very fact is the master key to unlocking our full potential. Because our world originates in our mind, we shape our existence by the type of thoughts that we allow to dominate our consciousness. By addressing the higher qualities in us, we position ourselves for success by realizing the unique powers, skills, talents, and abilities we've been given. By deliberately making the best choices that our minds and hearts can conceive, we set ourselves for the most fulfilled and meaningful existence available to us in this given body at this given time.

The best part of growing up is coming to know yourself. You realize you no longer need to repeat past mistakes.

When we learn a new skill and continue to practice it, our brain cells establish connections that solidify that new activity in our muscle memory and in our body. That's how later on we can do that activity repeatedly without paying attention to it. The flipside of this is that to unlearn a habit that's become ingrained in us we have to demolish that network of connections between our brain cells to train our mind and body into better activities. And following this principle, it means that at the beginning of this process of acquiring a new habit we have to pay close attention and be very diligent to repeat this new skill as frequently as possible until it becomes "stamped" into our mind and body (that is, muscle memory). This way, we trigger plastic changes in our brains that help it to rewire (reorganize) itself.[1]

The most effective and durable way to do that is by starting to practice a new activity that gives us pleasure. This can be physical pleasure or mental pleasure that is recognized as a positive activity that's good for us.

When we come to substitute new habits for the old ones it is critical to build an environment that is as positive and pleasurable as possible around this new good activity. This helps to create an entire new ecosystem of this positive new activity to be planted in our mind and body. It also releases dopamine, a reward chemical in the brain that induces excitement and good feelings. Dopamine is called the reward transmitter because when we accomplish something, for example, run and win a race, our brain triggers its release. We get a surge of energy, pleasure, and confidence, which further cements this positive new consciousness into the entire system of our mind and body. This way, you come to recognize this new habit on several levels: physically, because you've laid new circuits in your brain and it makes your body feel good; mentally, because you're aware that you're doing something that is good for you; and holistically, because you see that you are substituting an old bad habit for a good one that will last you for the rest of your life.

To state the obvious, this process can't be rushed. Remember this: When you cut corners, you shortcut yourself.

Society and popular culture might send you signals that in your fifties, sixties, and seventies you are too old and are supposed to not be able to change your habits. As we have seen repeatedly, that type of thinking is outdated and wrong.

One of the most important lessons you can take from this book is that you have a choice. You can choose to be rigid, be set in your ways, and not accept other points of view, or even not accept the premise that you have a choice. Or you can see yourself as a flexible, open-minded, creative person that neuroplasticity clearly shows that each person is capable of being.

The future is vast, open, and malleable. If you look at it correctly, the best years of your life can be ahead of you. This is a simple fact—if we make it so.

Neuroplasticity studies reveal that every single activity that we practice on a regular basis, whether physical, mental, or combining both those elements, changes both our brain and mind. Mentally, repetition and high concentration on that action cause the brain to develop and solidify connections between its cells to the point that it becomes "second nature" to us and we are able to practice it without effort. At the same time, the physical component of this mechanism develops muscle memory in the body, to the point where we're able to do this activity without applying much thought to it. The body remembers how to do it. Regular runners and swimmers know this system well. Once you begin the activity, the "autopilot" takes over—the arms are rowing, the lungs are pumping, the legs are kicking—and you can go in this manner for as long as your conditioning allows.

Brain scans have shown that every new skill we learn significantly modifies both the structure and behavior of the brain. We train our brain every time we develop a new ability. In essence, our present activities create the brain that we will have in the future. This is a result of the brain's plasticity throughout our entire life, and the foundation for our ability to replace past habits with new ones. Our brain's capacity to reorganize itself does not stop in our twenties, or thirties, or sixties. It goes on for as long as we live.[2]

Quitting Smoking

The single most important step you can take to help you quit cigarettes is to decide that you are ready to stop smoking now. This statement might seem obvious on its face value, but it contains in it a fundamental truth about overcoming nicotine addiction: Long-term smoking habits consists of both physical and mental dependence, and the process of freeing yourself of this addiction also needs to involve both your mind and body. You need to be at a place where you're tired of how smoking makes you feel, smell, and look, and are ready to make significant changes in your physical behavior and daily routines.

This is written from personal experience: Twenty-eight years ago I quit a fifteen-year habit of smoking a pack to a pack and a half a day. I initially quit cold turkey and stayed off cigarettes for eight months. At that point, thinking that I'd kicked the addiction, I lit a cigarette—and then smoked for another six months. This made me really disappointed in myself and at that time I quit again. However, every six months or so I would get an urge to light a cigarette with a drink, after a meal, or at a social gathering, and I would light up, and after the first few puffs my head would start spinning and I would get woozy, and this would remind me why I'd stopped putting this poison in my body. I haven't craved a cigarette for more than a decade, but this is also due to the active, healthy lifestyle I've been practicing, which helps me keep all addictions at bay.

In this chapter we use the term *let go,* because this is what you want to do: release from your body and mind the dependence you have on cigarettes by coming to realize that you don't need them for survival. Your body needs food and liquids to survive, but it doesn't depend on nicotine to exist. When we are born, this need is not a part of our genetic program. Because nicotine is not a vital substance in your life, you will learn how to expel it from your body and not have to rely on it for the rest of your life.

By now, the risks of smoking are well established and widely known. As noted in Chapter 10, a lifelong smoking habit cuts on average 10 years off a person's potential life span. On the other hand, even if you've been a heavy smoker for years, the benefits of quitting now are both enormous and immediate. After one month, the worst withdrawal symptoms subside and blood circulation in the body begins to improve steadily. Three months after quitting, lung function increases; at one year after quitting, excess risk of coronary heart disease drops to about half that of a smoker. At five years, lung cancer death rate for someone who had smoked a pack a day decreases by almost half. At ten years after quitting, risk of cancer of the mouth, throat, bladder, and kidney decreases significantly, and lung cancer death rate drops to that of nonsmokers. At fifteen years, risk of coronary heart disease is similar to that of people who have never smoked.[3]

Pressure points, ring muscles, and touch triggers are very effective tools to begin releasing the hold that nicotine has sprouted in your body. Ring muscle exercises will restore the original unified operation of the different systems in your body, which will enable the body to gradually eject this foreign invader; pressure-point routines will help you diffuse the cravings that you'll inevitably feel when you wean yourself off smoking; and touch triggers will enable you to plant new realization in your body that you don't need nicotine in your life.

Exercise: Using Psychosomatic Tools to Quit Smoking

The contractions and releases of the ring muscles stimulate a better blood flow in the body. This in turn boosts your body's overall vitality and loosens the roots that nicotine has grown in your system. (Revisit Chapter 9 to refresh your memory about the effects that pressure points, ring muscles, and touch triggers have in helping your body operate in its optimal condition.)

Just like your breath is a straight pathway into your inner core, so the pressure points of the body are direct doorways into the neural networks. Pressure points help expel nicotine dependence from your body by clearing up the passages between the different nerve centers in your body. This restores the body to its original state of not needing nicotine for its basic operation.

In addition to ring muscles, pressure points, and touch triggers, breathing exercises will help you throughout the day to deal with initial cigarette cravings and to regulate your body's energy by diverting your focus away from smoking onto the healthy and clean center you're establishing in yourself.

At the beginning, it is recommended to set aside at least 30 minutes daily for this exercise. The more time and attention you devote to this process the more you'll feel in control of overcoming your nicotine addiction.

Lie or sit down to the ring muscles session in your favorite place and begin a steady pattern of contractions and releases.

Make sure that your breathing is free, effortless, and deep.

Once you've established a comfortable routine of ring muscles, you will add pressure points to this exercise.

Using your thumb, forefinger, and middle finger gently begin applying pressure in your lower forehead just above the eyebrows. Lightly circle and massage the middle of your forehead, while breathing deeply into the place where your fingers touch your skin. Notice how tensions start escaping your body as you continue to softly rub your forehead.

Following the flow of your energy, you can move from your lower forehead to your eye sockets, and under your earlobe, where it meets the jaw and the neck. These places are extremely sensitive areas in your body because they're part of your nervous grid. By activating these network switches, you are relaxing the knots that nicotine has formed along your neural pathways. You help this process by exhaling deeply as these toxic deposits loosen their grip on your body. As you go about your day, whenever you feel cigarette craving coming on, you can diffuse this urge with a series of pressure points.

You can also add a touch trigger to help you quit smoking. For example, rubbing your knee or any other accessible spot in your body, while telling yourself, "I don't need this poison in my body, I don't need this poison in my body." As simple as that. You plant this new awareness in that spot in your body that you have no need for nicotine to survive. This is another tool in your toolkit to help rid yourself of smoking. The more tools you have, the better your chances of quitting.

The Mindful Breathing exercise (in Chapter 10) is also a good tool to use during the day, because it helps you manage the uneasy feelings you will experience at the beginning of withdrawal. It will also help to balance and align your body with free flow of energy.

You can do these exercises until you feel confident that nicotine has loosened its grip on your system. However, as we said about letting go of bad habits and acquiring good ones, we cannot leave a vacuum in our mind-body and lifestyle routines where that bad habit had been. This space needs to be filled with good and healthy activities instead.

We saw in Chapter 5 that our consciousness modulates our biology. Our thoughts affect our genes and not the other way around. Mind controls the body. Thoughts create new synapses—new connections—between our brain cells, and by repetition these new synapses, like strong branches of a tree, grow into thicker pathways between those particular neurons, which translate into a developed behavior that becomes a habit.

If your condition allows, choosing the more strenuous physical activities at the beginning, such as running, swimming, or tennis, will be more beneficial, because they will help your body cleanse the nicotine deposits in your lungs faster. But any physical activity you take up will help you substitute the fresh consciousness of well-being for the old residue of nicotine in your body.

In terms of lifestyle choices, this will require of you to begin changing the past behaviors that you associated with smoking, such as drinking, watching television, or following a meal with a cigarette, to new healthy habits that will keep your mind and body away from the need to smoke. It will help you replace each old bad habit with a good one in a fun and comfortable manner. Be creative: How about jumping rope for five to ten minutes after a meal to quench your need for a cigarette? Maybe a walk around the building or further away in your neighborhood? If you're up to it, perhaps a set of push-ups or jumping jacks? To reiterate, the idea is to do simple activities without needing to go out of your way. You can join a gym, but it's not essential to kick smoking and be in good shape. You can do it right here and now, in your immediate environment.

It's important to not be too harsh on yourself during this process. Remember the natural learning curve we discussed, in which episodic lapse into the old habit is par for the course. Recall the image of tango: two steps forward and one step back. The benefit of acquiring good new habits in place of the old negative ones is that once we repeat these new behaviors long enough, they become our new standard operation. New connection patterns are created in our brain to put in place of the old, and these new habits become the new norm.

It's not easy but it's doable. Many others have quit smoking and so can you. Be good to yourself and approach this process with small, gradual increments (the train ride mental imagery sequence is a great example), understanding that every day you live without a cigarette takes you farther away from harming your body and shortening your life toward a longer and healthier existence.

CHAPTER FIFTEEN

Creating Happiness

Just as the universe knows how to exist, so our body knows how to be healthy. Our job is to not harm the body with bad habits, which impair its ability to heal itself.

Your body contains a finite amount of energy. By now you have established a master structure in your life—a framework by which you know how long you could live if you make the right decisions. You have filled this scaffolding with your overriding philosophy of life—your creed. You have fit in your goals, dreams, ambitions, principles, and other essential values that are dear to you. All the beautiful future events you are imagining for yourself and your loved ones are also contained in this mental structure.

You are in the driver's seat, headed in the direction you've set for yourself. Keep in mind that reaching your destination is not the holy grail of your adventure. Rather, you need to reach your destination, whatever it may be, in the best condition you can be at that point—not out of breath, exhausted, and without friends, but healthy, happy, and surrounded by your loved ones. The analogy is to scaling Mount Everest. It's a great accomplishment, but your job is not yet done. For the successful end of the mission, you need to come down alive and unharmed.

This is where the mastery of all our available resources begins. Our resources are our various assets: intelligence, courage, heart, the energy in our body, our special talents, family relations, financial wealth, physical health, and every other attribute that makes us this unique individual. Your growing wisdom manifests itself in the way you manage and distribute your finite amount of energy over the entire framework of your life: how you master your passions, overcome your fears, harness your strengths and gifts, and navigate the challenging grid of life in an elegant manner. Keep in mind that sometimes the greatest enjoyment of life consists in doing something seemingly trivial (eating a bowl of fruit, taking a bath, going for a ride, watching a movie, or taking a nap). These, too, you'll miss when you're gone.

Our overall well-being is measured by the balance we create among our mind, body, and spirit. The human body is a well-organized system with a built-in mechanism to correct, repair, and regularly reset itself to its optimal condition. Rather than trying to enhance the body's natural operations with surgery or supplements, it is helpful to think of the process of healthy living as simply getting out of the body's way to let it do its job, by first not polluting it with harmful substances such as drugs and preservatives, and second, creating the optimal conditions of rest and good nutrition where the body can function in the manner it was designed.

Meaningful Existence

Even if our body is in its optimal condition, most people would feel that their existence is less than perfect if they don't feel a sense of meaning in their lives. It can be said that we humans are midway between animals and angels. Some people lean more toward one end than the other, but the human psyche contains the capacities for both. Searching for and finding meaning in existence separates humans from other forms of life. It is a crucial ingredient in what is considered by most people as life worth living.

Every life is unique, and finding meaning in one's existence is ultimately each individual's personal privilege and responsibility. If your current life feels out of balance, this means that you need to make the necessary changes that will get you back on track. Try to see this as an opportunity to grow and learn new things about yourself. Choose your favorite relaxation routine and a peaceful environment where you won't be disturbed, get writing materials (pen and paper, your smartphone, a tablet), make yourself comfortable, follow your breath into your center, and ask the most sincere and private questions of yourself:

- Why am I unhappy?
- What is missing in my life?
- Why do I feel out of balance?
- Why is there no meaning and a sense of satisfaction in my life?
- What is truly and deeply important to me in existence?
- Why is this important?
- What am I trying to accomplish by this?
- Am I honestly doing what I want to do?
- Am I the person that I dreamed I could be?
- What would excite me and make me feel that I'm living an authentic life that motivates me to be my best?
- What can I do that would bring out of me the finest qualities I have?

Ask these and other private questions of yourself, and when the answers come, write them down. Prioritize these answers in a descending order of importance: what is absolutely critical in your life, second most important, third, and so on. The purpose of this sincere personal inquiry is to pinpoint the source of your malaise. This is an essential step to enable you to correct the situation. This is not an easy practice, and it requires honesty, humility, courage, and patience. But this process also carries in it enormous promise of you uncovering in yourself vast resources of strength and vitality that will support your future life.

Humility can be your greatest strength. It distills your soul to its essence.

When you are given an ambition you're also given the means to accomplish it. This is how the universe operates through you. However you perceive your creator, whether it's a religious God, scientific Self-Organizing Dynamics, or a spiritual Source, it wants you to have the most fulfilling experience of existence. That is why it has created you. Moreover, it has given you those special dreams because it wants these visions brought forward in the world. These dreams are your individual mission in life. And you were given this particular mission because you have the tools to see it through.

When we're aligned with our purpose, our body resonates with health, energy, and life. Unfortunately, the opposite is also true. A recent study by the Centers for Disease Control and Prevention noted that there's an emotional component in 85 percent of illnesses.[1] Though it's important to acknowledge the legitimate benefits of medications in treating diseases, it's equally vital to recognize that in our quick-fix culture driven by the financial interests of Big Pharma, the natural challenges and tribulations of life (anxiety, sadness, grief, worry) have been made into pathological disorders. The pharmaceutical industry has created disfunctions where previously it was simply nature taking its course. They came up with a label for a condition and started advertising their solution for this "disorder." This way, normal trials of life have been made into mental and physical ailments (for example, short attention span, excess weight, lasting pain, anxiety, and age-related process in men [or, in pharma speak, erectile disfunction]).

This leads to seeing mental and physical illness where there is just normal human struggle. We can become so influenced by this brainwashing of commercials and marketing that we start thinking that simply having challenges in our life is a sign that there's something wrong with us. Needless to say, every medication has side effects, which upset the natural balance of the body. This profligate cycle of relying on drugs for every condition and easy access to prescriptions has led to the current opioid addiction epidemic in America, killing roughly 64,000 people in 2016, more than car accidents or guns.[2]

Life is not a beer commercial, in which everyone is happy and sexy all the time. Life can contain difficulties, heartbreak, disappointments, and pain. These are also part of being alive, and if we are to stay healthy and well-adjusted, we must accept and embrace these facts. We can't reduce existence into expecting it will always be comfortable and carefree. It is only through challenges that true growth happens. If we examine this in depth, we see that it can't be otherwise. When we are living a cushy contented existence, life does not require of us to search for hidden strengths; we are just cruising along. But when we face an unexpected challenge, that's when we are compelled to look for extraordinary powers. This is the time to discover the resources of wisdom and strength inside you.

You can do anything you want and anything you do has consequences. You make countless choices every day and these choices come to define you. As we have seen in neuroplasticity, the secret to our well-being lies in how we think. How we think determines every aspect of our life, big and small. It is helpful and fun to have little mantras to carry in your mental toolkit and use them as guideposts in your daily life. Instead of "mind over matter," think of "mind in harmony with matter." This implies understanding our mind and this particular body we have at present, and creating the daily conditions where we can be at our best both physically and mentally.

When we understand what we are, we see that we are limitless. When we understand and respect the basic laws of nature, we can do anything we desire.

Happiness Formula

To reiterate a point made earlier, every person is a distinct individual and there are hardly one-size-fits-all prescriptions when it comes to human affairs. However, there are concepts that research shows can apply to the vast majority of individuals. Social scientists who study happiness have developed the following formula: $H = S + C + V^3$.

H: Happiness =
S: Set point +
C: Conditions of living +
V: Voluntary actions

S = Set Point in our Brain

Unhappy people have a low set point because of their upbringing and past life events, and that influences their every experience. No matter what situation they face, they see the negative side of things, they complain, criticize, and see themselves as the victim. Happy people follow the Chinese proverb that says every crisis is a potential opportunity.

Can we change our set point? Yes.

Every time we see a challenge or a problem, we ask ourselves, "What's the opportunity here?"

Meditation is also a good way to change our set point. By taking a step back and reviewing the event from a cool distance, we can see how we might approach the situation differently.

Being mindful also changes our set point. This means not acting in a pre-conditioned manner, in a thoughtless manner, but instead asking ourselves, why do I want this? Why do I do this? Where will this lead me?

Set point accounts for about 45 percent of our happiness experience.

C = Conditions of Living

If we are very poor, it affects our level of happiness because then we think about money all the time. Studies find that what the poorest people and the richest people have in common is that they both constantly think about money. On the other hand, being very rich doesn't guarantee happiness. Research shows that the happiness level in people who have won the lottery rises immediately and plateaus at about six months, and by the end of the year people are back to their original happiness level. Conditions of living are responsible for roughly 10 percent of happiness.

Economists Daniel Kahneman, a 2002 Nobel Laureate, and Angus Deaton, a 2015 Nobel Laureate, who did research on the economic factors of happiness, found that annual income of $75,000 is the ideal mark for happiness. Below that level, there isn't enough money to spend time on favorite activities and with friends. Above that income threshold, there's no marked difference in the level of happiness.[4]

V = Voluntary Actions

The remaining 45 percent of our happiness level depends on the voluntary choices we make every day. These fall into two main types of choices that people normally make. First is for personal pleasure, and in the U.S. these are shopping; food, drinking, and entertainment; and sex. These activities make people happy, but this happiness lasts only a few days and then the level of happiness goes back to the original set point.

The choices that make people happy for the long term are those that give fulfillment, meaning, and purpose to their lives; when they are able to express their creativity; and when they can make somebody else happy. The easiest way to do this is by showing someone the three As: attention, affection, and appreciation.

It is our life, and the choices are given. Whether we enjoy this moment or not, is up to us. We decide what to make of it, and if we decide to make it a pleasant one, this decision carries in it happiness for us and those around us.

AFTERWORD

This book stands on the shoulders of the books cited on these pages and many more. The insights in those books inspired the ideas in this. This book is part of the continuum of exploration of ourselves and the cosmos. We humans keep wondering whether in a universe of billions upon billions of stars and planets—which is expanding at an accelerating rate—it is possible that the only life form in existence is tucked away in a small galaxy called the Milky Way, which is one of approximately 400 billion other galaxies in the observable universe, on a tiny planet called Earth. The simple answer is that we don't know. Without self-satisfied chauvinism, according to our present knowledge, humankind is the most advanced intelligence existing in the world.

Human minds are the conduits of consciousness in the universe and, until further discovery, human intelligence serves as the intelligence of the cosmos. Unified theory reveals that what is out there is also what's in here: that the structure of the macrocosm is identical to the structure of the microcosm. The human body is made according to and governed by the fundamental laws of nature. The more we understand ourselves the more we understand the universe, and vice versa. Evolution implies a growing awareness of ourselves and the cosmos.

If this book had been written five years ago, we could not have discussed many of the things we did on these pages. The recent discoveries simply were not available. And if we meet five years hence, we will know a lot more about ourselves (for example, further insights on how our brains work) and we'll have a better view of the distant edges of the cosmos, thanks also to the James Webb Space Telescope, expected to launch in spring 2019 and part of NASA's next-generation space telescope program. Evolution never stops.

We have covered in this book the developmental thresholds that humankind has passed since the big bang to the present, and where we might go from here. We can't reasonably say that we have reached the end of our progress as a species. Locating in ourselves the perception of our optimal duration is another small, important step in our continuous exploration of the amazing instrument of our mind-body-spirit. If we aim to be less than we're capable of being, we will probably never be happy.

What does sensing our optimal duration finally mean? It is like installing a fuel gauge in our vehicle of flesh, blood, and bones. Sensing your optimal duration of existence is another way of saying that you understand how much gas you have in your tank. This gives you more control over your vehicle and your destination, and enables you to go through life with knowledge.

If knowledge is power, lack of knowledge is lack of power. Can we exist without this perception as our predecessors did before the taming of fire or the invention of flying, and as early automobiles ran without fuel gauges? Does this cognition improve our daily lives? Clearly, because it gives us a more significant understanding of ourselves and of existence.

Let's recap the most immediate applications of this awareness in our daily lives. Seeing our optimal duration:

- Provides a framework for our life. When we are able to see the entire structure of our life we are better able to deal with the everyday challenges we confront.

- Gives us a healthy psychological distance from which to deal with periodic setbacks. On your larger journey of existence, this is where you are at present. Pace yourself.
- Gives us a sense of clarity, because we've seen the parameters of our life.
- Gives us stability, of knowing what we can control (our own thoughts and actions) and what is beyond our control, so we don't have to waste our energy worrying about it.
- Gives us confidence, in knowing that the power over our destiny and direction in life is in our hands.
- Leads to a sense of balance and internal peace, because it helps us understand the body that we inhabit and its proper relationship to our mind and spirit.

Seeing our finite time in the world prompts us to discover special value in each presumed remaining day.

It enables us to overcome the fear of death—because we've seen the fullness of our life.

It helps us manage anxieties and avoid desperate actions, because we can see our current setbacks in perspective.

And finally, seeing the entire arc of our journey enables us to fully realize our lifespan potential.

You are everything that the world knows up to this point. You are the product of evolutionary processes that have been taking place in the universe for the past 13.7 billion years since the big bang. This is the information that pulses through your bloodstream and animates your heartbeat.

Just as superstring theory shows that the universe is made of infinite packets of vibrating strings of potential that freeze into particular existence according to the observer and the type of intention being directed at them, so there are numerous forms of each individual existing as different potentials, and we bring into existence the best version of ourselves by the distinctive choices we make in our daily lives.

The capacity to sense your optimal duration gives you an enhanced way of managing life. However, as with other latent capacities we individually possess, such as having a talent for a musical instrument, a knack for languages, or being gifted in a particular sport, the inherent ability is only the promise of greatness: It needs to be nurtured with attention and practice.

This book listed many practical applications (body consciousness techniques, self-management skills, and mental imagery tools) to help you deal competently with life's different scenarios. I recommend that you select from among them the methods and guidelines that have resonated with you the most to carry in your mental toolkit for easy access throughout the day.

As you grow more familiar and confident with these exercises you will be able to combine some of them together into a personal routine—for example, meditating while you walk, jog, swim, or ride your bike; doing touch triggers on your way to the grocery as you use the mental imagery of an hourglass to deal with a challenge you're currently facing; doing pressure points to relieve stress while you're at your desk at work, watching television at home, or doing them discretely while riding a bus; doing a breathing exercise in combination with a touch trigger while lying in bed reading; or climbing the stairs as you regulate your breath and use a pressure point at the same time. The idea is that you gradually devise your own set of exercises that fit comfortably in your daily life and that make you feel healthy, vital, and balanced. After a while this will become your natural state of being. You will instinctively create the conditions that enable you to live your longest and healthiest life, according to the same principle: Listen to your body and trust it. Your body knows.

The great philosopher of fifth century BC, Socrates, wrote many wise things but when he said, "One thing I know is that I don't know anything," he was wrong. We can assume that he was speaking metaphorically because we can see that on the face of it, this statement is obviously false. Why?

Do you know pain? Do you know what makes you distraught, unhappy, and tense? Of course. Then you also know that you don't like pain, and you've probably learned how to avoid it. This is not insignificant.

We know hatred and we prefer love. We know strife and we prefer peace. We know chaos and we choose order. We know loneliness and we prefer the company of loved ones. These are not negligible things. These are the building blocks of a good and meaningful life.

We're not omnipotent. We acknowledge that in the universe there are forces much larger than ourselves, but this is no reason for us to feel helpless. Because we know pain we also know pleasure. Because we know illness we also know wellness. You know what it means to be healthy and what makes you happy, and you know what it feels like to love and be loved. You know compassion, and excitement, and curiosity, and self-awareness, and fulfillment (however you define it for yourself). These are not trivial issues. They are the fabric and the foundations of a life worth living. And they are in our hands.

From Buddha to Socrates to Hegel to Einstein to current breakthroughs in neuroscience and cosmology, we are doing now what we've always done: pushing the boundaries of darkness, ignorance, and dependence, to acquire knowledge, consciousness, and mastery over our lives and our surroundings.

It is good to remember that our thoughts affect our genes and not the other way around. You don't need to see yourself as declining in health as you age. Rather, you're making choices that enable you to be the best version of yourself at every age.

Our essence is eternal, but while we are in this lifetime, mastering our optimal duration leads to a more graceful existence.

NOTES

Chapter 3

1. "Jeanne Louise Calment: The World's Oldest Person," Department of Statistics—UC Davis website, *http://anson.ucdavis.edu/~wang/calment.html.*

Chapter 4

1. Krauss, Lawrence M. *A Universe from Nothing* (New York: Atria Books, 2012), p. 92.

2. Clara Moskowitz, "What's 96 Percent of the Universe Made of? Astronomers Don't Know," *www.space.com/11642-dark-matter-dark-energy-4-percent-universe-panek.html,* May 12, 2011.

3. Krauss, *A Universe from Nothing,* p. 89.

4. Moskowotz, "What's 96 Percent?"

5. Ibid.

6. NASA, "Hubble Reveals Observable Universe Contains 10 Times More Galaxies Than Previously Thought," October 13, 2016.

7. Krauss, *A Universe from Nothing*, p. 62.

8. Ibid., p. 106.

9. "Scientific Evidence that You Are Not the Body," The Science of Identity Foundation website, *www.scienceofidentityfoundation.net/yoga-philosophy /yoga-view-of-the-self/scientific-evidence-that-you-are-not-the-body.*

10. Scienceandnonduality. "What Is Consciousness? - Deepak Chopra, Rudolph Tanzi, Menas Kafatos and Lothar Schäfer," published November 13, 2013, 49:06, *www.youtube.com/ watch?v=scI9ZFImN8o.*

11. Krauss, *A Universe from Nothing*, p. 35.

12. ScienceNET. "7 Times Michio Kaku Went Next Level Genius," published January 30, 2017, 12:41, *www.youtube.com/ watch?v=BQn8dtla8BI.*

Chapter 5

1. Voytek, Bradley. "Are There Really as Many Neurons in the Human Brain as Stars in the Milky Way?" *Nature,* May 20, 2013.

2. Eagleman, David. *The Brain: The Story of You* (New York: Vintage Books, 2015), p. 190.

3. Ibid., pp.185–187.

4. Doidge, Norman, MD. *The Brain that Changes Itself* (New York: Penguin Books, 2007), p. 47.

5. "Bruce Lipton—The Power of Consciousness," Conscious.TV, transcript of interview by Iain McNay.

6. Ibid.

7. Doidge, *The Brain that Changes Itself*, p. 220.

8. "Jeanne Louise Calment."

Chapter 6

1. Salamanca, Alex. "25 Most Popular Animals on Google Search," List 25 website, *https://list25.com/25-most-popular-animals-on-google-search/,* updated May 15, 2015.

2. "List of Countries by Life Expectancy," Wikipedia, *https://en.wikipedia.org/wiki/List_of_countries_by_life_expectancy.*

3. Cohn, D'Vera, and Paul Taylor. "Baby Boomers Approach 65—Glumly," Pew Research Center, December 20, 2010, *www.pewsocialtrends.org/2010/12/20 /baby-boomers-approach-65-glumly/.*

4. Christensen, Kaare, Gabriele Doblhammer, Roland Rau, and James W. Vaupel. "Aging Populations: The Challenges Ahead," *The Lancet, V*ol. 374, No. 9696 (October 3. 2009): 1196–1208.

5. Ibid.

6. Wheeler, Rachel. "We'll Live to 100—How Can We Afford It?" World Economic Forum white paper, May 2017.

Chapter 7

1. Krauss, *A Universe from Nothing,* p. 107.

Chapter 8

1. Eagleman, *The Brain,* p. 177.

2. Personal correspondence with the author, January 2018.

3. Eagleman, *The Brain,* p. 120.

4. Doidge, *The Brain that Changes Itself,* p. 213.

Chapter 9

1. McSpadden, Kevin. "You Now Have a Shorter Attention Span than a Goldfish," *Time, http://time.com/3858309/attention-spans-goldfish/,* May 14, 2015.

Chapter 10

1. Quoi, Charles Q. "Is There a Limit to the Human Life Span?" LiveScience website, *www.livescience.com/59645-no-limit-to-human-life-span.html,* June 28, 2017.

2. Norton, Amy. "Depression Can Shave a Decade or More off Average Lifespan," *Health Day News,* October 23, 2017.

3. "Breathing Can Extend Lifespan by Several Decades," *The Onion,* 5 October 2017.

4. Jabr, Ferris. "Does Thinking Really Hard Burn More Calories," *Scientific American, www.scientificamerican.com/article/thinking-hard-calories/,* July 18, 2012.

5. Goldschmidt, Debra. "The Great American Sleep Recession," CNN, *www.cnn.com/2015/02/18/health/great-sleep-recession/index.html,* June 23, 2017.

6. Hafner, Marco, Martin Stepanek, Jirka Taylor, et al. "Why Sleep Matters—the Economic Costs of Insufficient Sleep: A Cross-Country Comparative Analysis," RAND Europe, 2016.

7. Ibid.

8. Nobel Prize press release, "The Nobel Prize in Physiology or Medicine 2017," *www.nobelprize.org/nobel_prizes/medicine/laureates/2017/press.html,* October 2, 2107.

9. Lee, I-Min, Eric J. Shiroma, Felipe Lobelo, Pekka Puska, Steven N. Blair, and Peter T. Katmarzyk. "Effect of Physical Inactivity on Major Non-Communicable Diseases Worldwide: An Analysis of Burden of Disease and Life Expectancy," *The Lancet, www.thelancet.com/journals/lancet/article/PIIS0140-6736(12)61031-9/fulltext,* July 18, 2012.

10. Doidge, *The Brain that Changes Itself,* p. 251.

11. Ibid.

Chapter 12

1. Choi, "Is There a Limit?"

2. Murphy, Michael. *The Future of the Body* (New York: Tarcher/Putnam, 1992), pp. 28–29.

3. Doidge, *The Brain That Changes Itself.*

4. Ibid., p. 3.

5. Eagleman, *The Brain,* p. 184.

6. Doidge, *The Brain That Changes Itself.*

7. Dossey, Larry. *The Extraordinary Healing Power of Ordinary Things* (Harmony Books, 2007).

Chapter 14

1. Doidge, *The Brain that Changes Itself,* p. 116.

2. Ibid., pp. 288–293.

3. "Stop Smoking Recovery Timetable," WhyQuit.com, *http://whyquit.com/whyquit/A_Benefits_Time_Table.html.*

Chapter 15

1. Mercola, Dr. Joseph. "E-motion—How Your Emotional Baggage May Be Sabotaging Your Health, and What to Do about It," Mercola.com, *https://articles.mercola.com/sites/articles/archive/2015/03/14/trapped-emotional-energy.aspx,* March 14, 2015.

2. Salam, Maya. "The Opioid Epidemic: A Crisis Years in the Making," *New York Times,* October 26, 2017.

3. Frankel, Mark. "The Happiness Formula H=S+C+V," Brevedy website, *www.brevedy.com/2013/12/18/the-happiness-formula-h-s-c-v/,* December 18, 2013.

4. "Happiness Economics," Wikipedia, *https://en.wikipedia.org/wiki/Happiness_economics.*

ACKNOWLEDGMENTS

This book has been 32 years in the making, and during that period there have been many good people who have contributed their time, attention, and advice to help bring it to publication.

I owe much gratitude to my capable and broad-minded agent, Marilyn Allen, whose natural curiosity won me over in our first conversation; she had me at "What are ring muscles?" My dear colleague Erantha De Mel, whose wise and kind energy run through every page of this book.

I thank the team of professionals at Career Press/New Page Books who welcomed this book into their roster: Michael Pye, for his kind, confident, and knowing guidance; Adam Schwartz, who shepherded the book through its initial steps in the publication process; Jeff Piasky, whose art direction and clear communication skills created the beautiful look of this book; talented cover designer Ian Koviak, who captured the spiritual and scientific essence of the manuscript; very talented editor Jodi Brandon, without whom the book would not be this clear and sharp. I'd like also to thank Laurie Kelly Pye, who added to the overall balance of the book.

Eryn Carter Eaton and Bonnie Hamilton, who generously gave of their knowledge and expertise to promoting the book. It's been a pleasure and honor to work with each one of them. I owe special thanks to Uwe Kind, who keeps inspiring me every day by how he lives and works. My good friend Eve Alintuck, who has given generously and continuously her valuable time and instruction. Greg Corbin, whose honest and generous notes made this book wiser and sharper. The formidable team of Scott Horstein and Antonia Glenn, for their critical and stimulating comments. And special acknowledgment is due to Rudolph Tanzi, who provided valuable insight from his research on intuition and also inspired the book's crowd-pleasing title.

I am deeply grateful to Esti Hen, Alik Asotsky, Ziva Simhi, John Camire, Ralph Proodian, Natallie Hen, Stephen Michaels, Joey Daigneault, Andrea Chase, and Israel Hen for their loving encouragement, and to the strong women in my life, Sarah, Hannah, and Manana, without whom none of this would be possible.

Lastly, and most importantly, my wife Teresa, whose intellectual and emotional support made this book simply more practical.

ABOUT THE AUTHOR

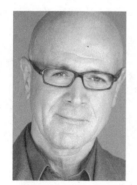 Guy Joseph Ale is the founding president of Lifespan Seminar and vice president of Asia Pacific Association of Psychology. He serves as the secretary general of the Chamber of Chartered Behavioral Scientists and is an Esteemed Council Member of the International Council of Professional Therapists.

Guy has earned a reputation as a visionary in the field of human life span. He received the Eminent in Psychological Science Award at the International Conference on Psychology 2011 "in recognition of invaluable contributions in the field of human lifespan." Lifespan Seminar received the Best of Beverly Hills Award in Health and Wellness Workshops, and the Los Angeles

Excellence Award in the Life Coach category, for the last four years in a row. In Hollywood, Guy is affectionately known as the "Life Coach for the Stars."

Guy lectures and conducts workshops in the United States, Europe, and Asia. Learn more at *www.LifespanSeminar.com.*